Sambadrama
The Arena of Brazilian Psychodrama

Edited and translated by Zoltán Figusch

Forewords by Adam Blatner and José Fonseca

Jessica Kingsley Publishers
London and Philadelphia

First published in 2006
by Jessica Kingsley Publishers
116 Pentonville Road
London N1 9JB, UK
and
400 Market Street, Suite 400
Philadelphia, PA 19106, USA

www.jkp.com

Copyright © Jessica Kingsley Publishers 2006
Foreword copyright © Adam Blatner 2006
Foreword copyright © José Fonseca 2006

All rights reserved. No part of this publication may be reproduced in any material form (including photocopying or storing it in any medium by electronic means and whether or not transiently or incidentally to some other use of this publication) without the written permission of the copyright owner except in accordance with the provisions of the Copyright, Designs and Patents Act 1988 or under the terms of a licence issued by the Copyright Licensing Agency Ltd, 90 Tottenham Court Road, London, England W1T 4LP. Applications for the copyright owner's written permission to reproduce any part of this publication should be addressed to the publisher.
Warning: The doing of an unauthorised act in relation to a copyright work may result in both a civil claim for damages and criminal prosecution.

The right of the contributors to be identified as authors of this work has been asserted by them in accordance with the Copyright, Designs and Patents Act 1988.

Library of Congress Cataloging in Publication Data

Sambadrama : the arena of Brazilian psychodrama / edited and translated by Zoltán Figusch; forewords by Adam Blatner and José Fonseca.
  p. cm.
Includes bibliographical references and indexes.
ISBN-13: 978-1-84310-363-9 (pbk. : alk. paper)
ISBN-10: 1-84310-363-X (pbk. : alk. paper)

 1. Psychodrama--Brazil. I. Figusch, Zoltán, 1974-
RC489.P7S26 2005
616.89'1523--dc22
                                    2005018962

British Library Cataloguing in Publication Data
A CIP record for this book is available from the British Library

ISBN-13: 978 184310 363 9
ISBN-10: 184310 363 X

Printed and bound in Great Britain by
Athenaeum Press, Gateshead, Tyne and Wear

*To Jussara,
for bringing me to Brazil*

Contents

FOREWORD BY ADAM BLATNER 9

FOREWORD BY JOSÉ FONSECA 10

ACKNOWLEDGEMENTS 11

INTRODUCTION 13

Part 1 The history and identity of Brazilian psychodrama 15

1 The arrival of psychodrama in Brazil: Its early development in the 1960s 17
Ronaldo Pamplona Da Costa

2 The development of psychodrama theory in Brazil 35
Sergio Perazzo

3 The roles of the colonized and the colonizer: In search of the identity of Brazilian psychodrama 48
José Fonseca

4 The role of the colonizer and the colonized: In search of the identity of Brazilian psychodrama 60
Geraldo Massaro

Part 2 Theoretical innovations in Brazilian psychodrama 69

5 The 'nucleus of the I' theory of Jaime Rojas-Bermudez 71
Zoltán Figusch

6 The clusters theory 90
Dalmiro M. Bustos

7 Digression around certain aspects of role theory 122
Sergio Perazzo

8	The protagonist and the protagonic theme Luís Falivene R. Alves	130
9	The theatre of spontaneity and psychodrama psychotherapy Moysés Aguiar	141

Part 3 Innovative techniques in Brazilian psychodrama   157

10	Psychogram: The use of drawings in psychodrama psychotherapy Luis Altenfelder	159
11	Genodrama: Psychodramatic work with genograms in couple therapy Maria Amalia Faller Vitale	175
12	Dramatic multiplication Pedro Mascarenhas	190
13	I hate you…please don't leave me!: The borderline client and psychodrama Rosa Cukier and Sonia Marmelsztejn	203
14	Sociometry: A new way to calculate the indices of the perceptive test Antonio Ferrara	227
15	Video-psychodrama and tele-psychodrama: The research of a Morenian dream Ronaldo Pamplona da Costa	250

APPENDIX: DIRECTORY OF THE PSYCHODRAMA ORGANIZATIONS AFFILIATED TO THE BRAZILIAN PSYCHODRAMA FEDERATION (FEBRAP)	268
REFERENCES	273
CONTRIBUTORS	278
SUBJECT INDEX	280
AUTHOR INDEX	285

Foreword

Psychodrama involves ideas and methods that have many applications in therapy and social development throughout the world. At present, Brazil has more psychodramatists than any other country. I've encouraged Zoltán Figusch, the editor of this book, to share the work of his colleagues. Readers will benefit from his selecting a broad spectrum of views and helping us to appreciate the diversity, originality, creative thinking, and depth of experience of respected practitioners and teachers of psychodrama in Brazil. Figusch's prodigious effort in translating their writings into English is a contribution to our field, and I hope it will inspire others in the international psychodrama community to consider doing the same. It is with gratitude that I welcome this book to the body of literature in psychodrama, sociometry and group psychotherapy.

Adam Blatner M.D., T.E.P., certified trainer in psychodrama, fellow of the American Psychiatric Association, certified psychiatrist, and author of Acting-In *and* Foundations of Psychodrama.

Foreword

I see this book as a fundamental effort to create a bridge between the Brazilian and the international psychodrama community. Despite its voluminous literature (with over a hundred psychodrama books published in Portuguese), Brazilian psychodrama is hardly known in other parts of the world. By selecting and translating significant writings of the Brazilian psychodrama caucus, Zoltán Figusch breaks through the language barrier, offering international readers a wide and extensive view of our technical and theoretical innovations. While living in Brazil, Zoltán Figusch became an active member of our psychodrama movement and a tireless explorer of Brazilian psychodrama literature. This book is the result of his skilful selection of some of our most important writings. As a recognition of his achievement, I would like to see Zoltán Figusch become an ambassador for Brazilian psychodrama in the United Kingdom.

José Fonseca, M.D., Ph.D., São Paulo Psychodrama Society (SOPSP), DAIMON Centre of Relationships Studies

Acknowledgements

I would like to thank the authors of the various chapters for their contribution, enthusiasm and support, with special thanks to José Fonseca for welcoming me in Brazil, for his valuable suggestions and opinions and for allowing me to use his personal library while doing my research for this book. I would also like to thank Adam Blatner for his inspiring foreword, as well as Leonie Sloman and Ruth Ballantyne for their support on the editorial side. Last but not least, a big thank you to my wife Jussara, who helped me overcome my difficulties with the Portuguese language and supported me all along as I was working on this book.

Zoltán Figusch

Introduction

Beyond being the country of sunshine, football, the Carnival and samba, Brazil is also the home of the largest psychodrama community in the world, with the Brazilian Psychodrama Federation (FEBRAP) embracing as many as 4,000–5,000 practitioners and nearly 50 psychodrama organizations. Brazilian psychodramatists have also produced a very extensive literature, authoring around a hundred books and as many as a thousand articles published in various journals. However, since they are written in Portuguese, this valuable material has, until now, been unavailable, to English-speaking psychodrama professionals.

The idea of translating and editing a collection of Brazilian psychodrama writings first came to me when I read Adam Blatner's paper[1] in which he presents a brief history of the Brazilian psychodrama movement and calls for a translation of their best writings. Simple it may seem, but it was not an easy task! How could one select the 'best writings' from such an extensive literature? How could one even read through so many books and articles? It took me nearly a year of research to reach the point where I could draw up the first outline for the contents of this book. I have since reviewed this initial structure numerous times, and – as I still continuously come across many interesting new writings – even today I occasionally think that more chapters could have been included, or that other areas of the Brazilian psychodrama practise could have been presented. However, this book has its physical limitations and so I had to accept that there is only so much that can possibly be included here.

When trying to select the chapters for this book my intention was to present a fairly wide picture of the contributions made by Brazilian psychodramatists. This is why I have eventually divided the book into three main parts. Within the first part I present the historical background and the development of the Brazilian psychodrama movement, with a strong focus on its specific cultural identity. The second part covers Brazilian innovations and developments of the psychodrama theory, while the third part focuses on innovations in the technique and practise of psychodrama. In the expectation that not only will this material awaken the interest of English readers but that it will also lead to some dialogue and exchange of experiences, I have included in the Appendix a directory of Brazilian psychodrama organizations. I would like to see this book as a bridge for professional communication between psychodramatists of various countries and nationalities, and as a bridge across cultures, across the Northern and Southern hemispheres.

Why *Sambadrama*? One of Brazil's world famous attractions is the Carnival when every February, millions of people celebrate, dancing for days on end to the rhythm of samba. The arena where all this celebration takes place is called *sambódromo* in Portuguese (the English equivalent would be 'samba-drome'). Within the sambódromo, colourful, creative and beautiful scenes of Brazilian life, history and imagination unfold, as presented by the various samba schools. So, 'sambadrama' is a play upon words, an allusion to the Portuguese sambódromo; *Sambadrama* – the book – presents the scenes that unfold in the arena of Brazilian psychodrama. It is a collection of writings and papers describing the colourful and diverse scenery of this rich and fascinating psychodrama culture, aiming to bring the latest innovations in theory and practise to the English-speaking world, making these important discoveries available to the benefit of practitioners and clients across the globe.

All the chapters were written by experienced and leading Brazilian practitioners; when translating I tried to stay as faithful as possible to the original and to maintain the individual style of each author (in the Notes at the end of the chapters an asterisk marks my additional editor's note), preserving the specific flavour of each paper. However, as with selecting the 'best writings' of Brazilian psychodramatists, I can only hope that the English text has turned out as enjoyable as the original Portuguese ones are.

And now, let's samba!

Zoltán Figusch[2]

Note

1   Blatner, A. (2000) 'History of Psychodrama in Brazil', Brazilian Psychodrama Federation (FEBRAP), http://febrap.org.br/macro.asp
2   If you have any comments on this book or on Brazilian psychodrama, please email the editor at figusch@hotmail.com

Part 1

The history and identity of Brazilian psychodrama

Part 1 contains four chapters concerning the beginnings and the history of the psychodrama movement in Brazil, and the development of the Brazilian psychodrama identity.

The first chapter, by Ronaldo Pamplona Da Costa, is the first comprehensive account ever written that presents the various roots of Brazilian psychodrama in great detail – the historical background against which psychodrama appeared, took hold and started to develop in Brazil, striving towards its own national identity.

Sergio Perazzo continues the story of the Brazilian psychodrama movement, focusing on some of the most significant and relevant theoretical developments introduced by Brazilian psychodramatists.

The authors of the last two chapters within this section are in search of the identity of Brazilian psychodrama. José Fonseca discusses the roles of the colonizer and the colonized in the light of Moreno's 'role theory,' stressing the importance and necessity of finding a Brazilian identity within the areas of psychotherapy and psychodrama rather than imitating the techniques used by the colonizers. In the last chapter Geraldo Massaro also assesses some aspects of the colonization of Brazil. He considers psychodrama as a cultural product that has been 'imported' to Brazil, analysing how it adapted to the local social, cultural and political circumstances.

The history and identity of Brazilian psychiatry

1

The arrival of psychodrama in Brazil
Its early development in the 1960s[1]

Ronaldo Pamplona Da Costa

I have been involved with the psychodrama movement since 1970 and I actively took part in the development of the Psychodrama Remembrance Project[2] coordinated by Carlos Borba. Information gathered for this project helped me to trace back the first seeds of psychodrama that were planted in Brazilian soil. Another important source of information for this chapter was Montagna's (1994) account of the two forerunners of Brazilian psychodrama: the psychiatry and psychoanalysis practised in São Paulo within the first half of the twentieth century. These two movements were important because on the one hand, it was the psychiatrists who first introduced psychodrama into their medical institutions and, on the other hand, until the 1960s there was only one psychotherapeutic movement in Brazil: psychoanalysis. It was only in the 1960s that group psychotherapy appeared and made its first steps in Brazil; the development of this movement is going to be one of my other important references within this chapter. I will also make reference to the Sedes Sapientiae Institute from São Paulo, where Mother Cristina was promoting the 'opening of the harbours of psychotherapy'. And finally, I will write about the São Paulo Psychodrama Study Group, the first psychodrama institute in Brazil where, between 1968 and 1970, the first psychodrama courses were held by the Argentinean psychiatrist and psychodramatist Jaime Rojas-Bermudez.

My aim is to identify the different roots of Brazilian psychodrama that eventually led to the development of its present identity. I will mainly focus on the psychodramatic movement from São Paulo; the reason for this is that there is only very little information available regarding the development of psychodrama in Belo Horizonte, started in the 1960s by Pierre Weil and

Célio Garcia. Finally, with this chapter I would like to pay homage to both the foreign and the Brazilian pioneers of psychodrama.

Psychiatry and psychoanalysis in São Paulo in the first half of the twentieth century

In São Paulo, in the mid-nineteenth century the insane were confined together with the criminals in the 'Hospice of the Madman' (Hospício dos Alienados) and in the Várzea do Carmo Asylum. At that time both institutions were administrated by laymen.

In 1886 the Juqueri Hospice was founded by Dr Francisco Franco da Rocha (1864–1933), a psychiatrist influenced by the French humanistic ideas that Pinel introduced into psychiatry. In one of his books Franco da Rocha wrote: 'Madness will be overcome, when the founders of psychiatric asylums will try to surround the sick with physical conditions and moral influences that provide a more enlivening environment, a more peaceful and calm spirit, thus inhibiting the impulses of delirium.'

In his attempt to overcome and treat madness, Franco da Rocha combined different psycho-social therapies, among which he highlighted work-therapy. With the realization of his project, São Paulo became a leading centre of psychiatry.

In 1919, in the opening session of the psychiatry course at the São Paulo Medical School, Franco da Rocha delivered a lecture entitled 'Of the deliriums in general', in which, citing Freud he talked about the necessity of finding a new understanding of madness. He was already considered a pioneer by introducing work-therapy at the Juqueri Hospice, but proved to be innovative yet again when he published a work based on his research entitled 'The pansexualism of the Freudian doctrine'. These contributions marked the arrival of the dynamic perspective in Brazilian psychiatry.

For Durval Marcondes (1899–1981) – then a young student at the Medical School – Franco da Rocha's book meant his first encounter with psychoanalysis. Later on, he became a crucial figure in introducing the psychoanalytic movement in São Paulo.

In 1923 Franco da Rocha retired from Juqueri and his post was taken by Dr Antônio Carlos de Pacheco e Silva, a neuro-pathologist trained in France. He worked in a bacteriologist spirit (trying to find biological and physical causes for mental illness) characteristic of those times and established at Juqueri an era of organic research, with a focus on finding physical agents that are responsible for mental illnesses. Under the administration of Pacheco e Silva a laboratory of pathological anatomy, an X-ray department (for the scanning of the central nervous system) and the use of convulsive therapy developed. Pacheco e Silva stayed in his post for 15 years and was discharged in 1938.

In 1924, the freshly qualified Dr Durval Marcondes started a correspondence with Freud and signed up for the International Journal of Psychoanalysis. In the same year he initiated and taught the first psychoanalysis course in São Paulo (and the whole country). He was self-taught and through his studies he gained sufficient knowledge to practise psychoanalysis.

In 1926 Franco da Rocha retired from his teaching post at the Medical School, where he was also chair of the psychiatry section. The new candidate for the psychiatry cathedra was not approved, leaving the place fully to the disposition of a neurologist called Dr Enroljas Vampré, who for ten years became the chair of both the Psychiatry and Neurology sections.

Ten years later, in 1936, Pacheco e Silva and Marcondes both applied for the post of the psychiatry chair. The ensuing dispute developed into a clash between clinical psychiatry and psychoanalysis. With the victory of Pacheco e Silva a strong campaign started against psychoanalysis which became even more vehement when Pacheco e Silva became chair of psychiatry at the Paulista Medical School as well.

In the same year (1936) Adelaide Koch arrived in Brazil. She was a German doctor and an analytic trainer from the International Psychoanalytic Association (IPA) – founded by Freud. With the authorization of Dr Ernest Jones and Otto Fenichel, she became responsible for the training of the first Brazilian psychoanalysts, including Durval Marcondes, Darcy de Mendonça Uchôa, Flávio Dias and Virgínia Bicudo (Bicudo being the only one who wasn't a medical doctor).

Since he had started his own training courses, Durval Marcondes was continuously trying to get psychoanalysis recognized by the academic psychiatry caucus, but never succeeded. In 1927 Marcondes founded the Brazilian Psychoanalytic Society, which gathered 24 members, but did not manage to achieve what he intended: to lift psychoanalysis to a scientific status; a status that psychoanalysis had already achieved in Europe and the United States. A few years later the Brazilian Psychoanalytic Society was dissolved. Only the arrival of Koch made it possible for the Brazilians to have a training recognized by the IPA.

Already during the first training group a new proposal was suggested, namely that people without a medical background (at the time there were no psychologists) should also be allowed to become psychoanalysts, as was the case for Virgínia Bicudo. On 5 June 1944 the São Paulo Psychoanalytical Group was founded by Koch and other analysts trained by her. In 1951 their name changed to São Paulo Psychoanalytic Society and it received a definitive recognition from the IPA.

From the facts related above we can see that psychoanalysis did not receive the support of academic psychiatry, or more precisely, was not supported by the psychiatrists connected to the São Paulo Medical School and the Paulista Medical School. It was supported however, by the professionals from Juqueri, the Aché Institute and the Bela Vista Sanatorium, these latter two being private hospitals.

In the same year when the Paulista Medical School was founded (1933), a Superior Institute of Pedagogy, Science and Literature was also established by the Sisters of the 'Nossa Senhora Cônegas de Santo Agostinho' Congregation. From the 1960s (and up to the present day) this institute, from which later on the Sedes Sapientae Institute originated, became the home of psychodrama and numerous other psychotherapeutic movements. In 1940, Sister Célia Sodré Dória (Mother Cristina), who later became the director of the Institute, obtained a degree in philosophy and pedagogy and soon after went to Europe, where she completed her studies about Freud. In 1954 she obtained a doctorate in Educational Psychology at the Catholic University of São Paulo (PUC-SP).

Mother Cristina was born in 1916, and grew up in the middle of political discussions and learnt the importance of respect and love. The institution she directed was dedicated to the concretization of these two ideas: politics and psychology. In one of her talks she said: 'The Sedes Sapientae Institute is an open space for those who want to learn and put into practise a project for the transformation of our society, aiming to build a world where social justice is the highest law.' In 1954 the Institute opened its new, four storey Psychological Clinic, offering the study and practise of psychology for 375 students and planned to satisfy the needs of many more.

In the same year, the fourth-hundredth birthday of the City of São Paulo was commemorated, and among the several different scientific events organized for this occasion, the first Latin-American Health Conference also took place, organized by the São Paulo Medical Association.

In order to understand the importance and significance of this conference, we need to stress that from 1949 the International Movement of Mental Hygiene changed its name to World Health Organisation and since that time health was defined as 'a state of physical, psychological, mental and social well-being, which is not just simply the absence of an illness'. It was from this time onwards, that psychological well-being started to seek the support of psychoanalysis and other psychotherapeutic movements. The president of the above-mentioned 1954 conference was Pacheco e Silva, while Durval Marcondes was one of the vice-presidents. This resulted in a real confrontation between psychiatrists and psychoanalysts. The main issue was that psychiatrists did not want to accept psychoanalysts from a non-medical background.

Even though the academic psychiatrists have started to accept the practise of psychoanalysis, they did not necessarily approve of the analytic training and disapproved even more strongly of the training of non-professional analysts, with the argument that 'psychotherapy is for doctors'. However, psychoanalysis already had the support of numerous non-academic psychiatrists, who showed a strong interest in psychoanalysis. There were so many people applying for training at the São Paulo Psychoanalytic Society that it overwhelmed the capacity of the trainers. By 1950 there was a waiting list of 40 people (Montagna 1994).

Since psychoanalysis was the only available formal training in psychotherapy, many psychiatrists became interested in learning group psychotherapy. At that time many psychoanalysts also started to work with therapeutic groups. It is due to this fact that psychoanalytically-based group psychotherapy arrived in Brazil, and started to be practised in three different cities: São Paulo, Rio de Janeiro and Porto Alegre. Until the First Latin-American Conference of Group Psychotherapy (Buenos Aires, 1957) these three centres were developing in isolatation from each other. They were autonomous, their professionals self-taught and most of them analysts. At the Buenos Aires conference however, the professionals of these three cities had a chance to exchange their experiences, and it was this encounter that gave birth to the movement that further expanded during the 1960s and served as a fertile soil for the seeds of psychodrama.

In 1958 the first psychology course was set up at the São Paulo University. A year earlier the Catholic University of Rio de Janeiro (PUC-RJ) was founded. In 1962 psychology courses started at the Catholic University of São Paulo (PUC-SP) and the Sedes Sapientae Institute as well (Coimbra 1995).

Pierre Weil (a Belgian psychologist settled in Brazil) had, in the 1950s, already started to experiment with the use of psychodrama for managerial training (in Rio de Janeiro) (Weil 1967).

Even earlier than this, in 1949, a black sociologist called Guerriero Ramos presented a seminar on group psychotherapy, sociodrama and psychodrama at the National Institute of Black People, in Rio de Janeiro. At that time Ramos lived in the USA where he learnt psychodrama with Moreno and in 1950 he was the editor of the *Sociometry* journal (Oliveira 1990).

In 1957 Íris Soares de Azevedo, a sociology student at São Paulo University, met professor Otto Kleinberg,[3] and through this encounter she got in touch with Moreno's ideas. She was fascinated by the fact that Kleinberg was combining the theories of sociology and psychology. The following year Azevedo enrolled for a specialization course in clinical psychology at the Sedes Sapiantae Institute, but without any previous psychology training. At that time, any professional who wanted to work with psychotherapy patients had to complete this two-year long training in clinical psychology; up until 1958 this was the only way for professionals to train in psychology (Borba first video 1993).[4]

The pioneers of Brazilian psychodrama

The 1960s were politically disturbing times in Brazil; first the movements of the left and then the military coup of 1964 changed the history of the country, bringing to an end the democratic experience that started in 1946.

Although politically fateful for the democracy, the 1960s were also the decade of psychodrama in Brazil. The practise of psychodrama started in three different centres: São Paulo, Ribeirão Preto and Belo Horizonte; Íris Soares Azevedo being its pioneer in São Paulo, Dr Flávio D'Andrea in Ribeirão Preto, and Célio Garcia in partnership with Pierre Weil in Belo Horizonte.

Through the establishment of numerous private hospitals, psychiatry was facing a great expansion. The São Paulo Psychoanalytic Society (SPSP) became more consolidated but also more enclosed in itself (perhaps as a consequence of the 'persecution by the academic psychiatrists'), trying to make its membership more exclusive. Many of its members went to Europe to re-analyse and refine their theoretical knowledge.

There was a great demand for psychoanalytic training. There were around 70 professional candidates on the waiting list of the SPSP wanting to be trained in psychoanalysis (Montagna 1994). In São Paulo, by 1967 psychoanalytically-based group psychotherapy strengthened significantly, opening up the space for the development of psychodrama.

In 1960 the second Latin-American Conference of Group Psychotherapy was held in Santiago (Chile), where 24 Brazilians presented their work. In the same year Norma Jatobá (a psychologist) started to use psychodrama in her private practise, blending it with art-therapy. As part of her internship, Jatobá spent three years in Paris during the 1950s, where she worked together with other French psychodramatists. In the same year (1960) encouraged by Mother Cristina, Íris Azevedo also started her psychodrama practise (Borba first video 1993).

The year 1960 was also marked by another important event: the São Paulo Society of Psychology and Group Psychotherapy was founded, having as its president the psychoanalyst Bernardo Blay Neto.

In 1961 Célio Garcia (psychologist) started to run psychodrama groups for children and adolescents at the Medical-Pedagogical Centre in Belo Horizonte. He worked together with Lea Porto and Maria Célia de Castro Bessa as trained auxiliaries (Weil 1967).

At the Sedes Sapientae Institute (São Paulo) Azevedo was further encouraged in her psychodrama work by a child psychiatrist called Haim Gruspun, who studied psychodrama in Europe and worked at the Sedes Sapientae Institute at the time (Borba first video 1993).

Together with Ângelo Gaiarsa (psychopathology lecturer), Gruspun was teaching play-therapy within the Psychotherapeutic Techniques Course promoted by Mother Cristina at the Sedes Sapientae Institute. Besides the psychoanalytic training, this was the only available psychotherapy course at the time. Gaiarsa and Gruspun also worked as consultant therapists at the institute (Gruspun 1998).

In the same year (1961) Azevedo was invited by Paulo Guadêncio (psychiatrist) to work in his private office at the Honduras Clinic. Based only on their readings of Moreno's books, they started to run psychodrama groups with adolescents. Alfredo Soeiro and J.M. D'Alessandro were also employed as trained auxiliaries (Borba first video 1993).

In 1962 psychology was finally recognized as a profession by the Ministry of Education and Culture. In the same year, influenced by Moreno's book 'Who shall survive?', a newly qualified doctor called Flávio Fortes D'Andrea started to use psychodrama and sociometry at the psychiatric out-patient's department of the Ribeirão Preto Medical School. He managed to successfully treat numerous patients who did not respond to other forms of treatment available at the hospital. He was in correspondence with Moreno, who approved of his practise and also sent him articles and books. D'Andrea was the author of the first psychodrama article in Brazil, published in the São Paulo Medical Journal (1963). Moreno invited D'Andrea to become a member of the International Association of Group Psychotherapists (IAGP), a proposal that he accepted. D'Andrea became one of the first Brazilians to work with the Morenian method, and also the pioneer of introducing psychodrama in the training of medical psychiatry and nursing (D'Andrea 1985).

In 1963 the third Latin-American Conference of Group Psychotherapy was held in Rio de Janeiro, where 14 Brazilian psychoanalysts gave presentations. In the same year, a group of 13 group psychotherapists and psychoanalysts founded the Brazilian Association of Analytical Group Psychotherapy in São Paulo (Zimmermann 1971). In the same year, Íris Soares Azevedo ran five therapeutic psychodrama groups with adolescents in her private practise.

In the Medical-Pedagogical Centre of Belo Horizonte (today called the Psycho-Pedagogical Institute of Minas Gerais), Léa Porto continued the psychodrama work started by Célio Garcia, having Márcio Pacheco as trained auxiliary (Weil 1967). In São Paulo, Darcy Uchôa (a psychiatrist and psychoanalyst) became director of the Psychiatry Department of the Paulista Medical School, opening up new possibilities for the application of psychoanalysis within the academic realm in São Paulo. As part of his internship in psychoanalytic psychodrama, Antônio Carlos Cesarino spent six months in Paris, where he worked with Serge Lebovici (Borba first video 1993).

In 1964 the Fourth Latin-American Conference of Group Psychotherapy was held in Porto Alegre (Brazil), where 53 Brazilians presented their research, two of these carried out in the field of psychodrama by D'Andrea. This was the first time that a psychodrama work was presented at a medical conference organized in Brazil. At this conference Bermudez (an Argentinean psychodramatist) also directed a public psychodrama session. For the first time in Brazil, Moreno's method was presented in its most genuine form (a public psychodrama) within a medical conference.

The year 1965 was a quiet one for the developing Brazilian psychodrama field. Its pioneers – Azevedo, D'Andrea, Garcia and Weil – continued their work and development of psychodramatic research. It is important to mention that the three psychodrama centres had no contact with each other yet. D'Andrea published an article entitled 'Sociodrama as a dynamic tool in the diagnosis of hostility between groups', in the *Sociology* journal from São Paulo. A psychiatry department was set up at the São Paulo State Hospital, where D'Alessandro started to run psychodrama groups for adolescents. In Belo Horizonte, Pierre Weil set up a psychodrama theatre, where he worked with the triadic psychodrama learnt from Anne Ancelin in Paris (Borba sixth video 1998).

From 1966 Anne Ancelin started to make regular visits to Brazil, and together with Pierre Weil she gave seminars about the triadic psychodrama in Minas Gerais and Rio de Janeiro states. Professionals from São Paulo, however, had no knowledge of these seminars (Borba seventh video 1998).

In 1966, following the retirement of Pacheco e Silva from the São Paulo Medical School, the psychoanalytic practitioner Darcy Uchôa (who already held the Chair of Psychiatry at the Paulista Medical School) applied for the post together with Fernando Bastos. The post was given to Bastos who, while opposing psychoanalysis, started to open more and more space for psychodrama during the 1960s and 1970s (Montagna 1994).

The third International Psychodrama Conference was organized in Barcelona (Spain), and was attended by Azevedo, Soeiro, D'Alessandro and Carvalho. For the first time, this group of self-taught professionals who had already worked with psychodrama for seven years, had the chance to see Moreno, Zerka and Bermudez direct. According to Azevedo, the way Bermudez was working seemed to be closer to Brazilian culture. After returning to Brazil she was invited by the psychiatry department of the São Paulo Hospital to report on her experiences from the conference (Borba first video 1993). She realized that in São Paulo, where until then only individual psychoanalysis, group psychotherapy and (Mother Cristina's) dynamic psychotherapy were practised, psychodrama had started to get more and more attention as a new psychotherapeutic method. Psychodrama however, was also considered a technique of the hysterics, as a possibility of 'acting-out'. At the hospital Azevedo was introduced with slight indifference to Dr Clóvis Martins, director of the psychiatry department. It is possible that the explanation for this disregard was manifold: she was a woman (the ideas of feminism had barely arrived in Brazil at the time), she was a psychologist (a profession that, legally speaking, was non-existent), and she was proposing an action method (psychoanalysis proposes inaction). According to Oswaldo Di Loreto, in those years, psychodrama was seen as some sort of curiosity, similar to how people relate nowadays to alternative therapies (Borba thirteenth video 1986).

In 1967 the first book written in Portuguese was published about the Morenian methodology. It was entitled 'Psychodrama', its author was Pierre Weil with a foreword by J.L. Moreno.

The first public psychodrama session in São Paulo

In May 1967 the fifth Latin-American Conference of Group Psychotherapy was held in São Paulo, organized by the São Paulo Society of Psychology and Group Psychotherapy (Zimmermann 1971).

The significance of this conference was that it represented the definite introduction of psychodrama in São Paulo. Seventy Brazilians presented papers on group psychotherapy. Among them were many who were later to become students of Bermudez: Carol Sonnenreich, Jeni Coronel Lustosa, Miguel Navarro, A.C. Eva, José Fonseca, A.C. Cesarino, Anibal Mehzer, Zacaria Ramadan, Maria Aleuda Moreno, José S.M. Werneck. Many psychoanalysts also attended the conference. It became clear that verbal group psychotherapy had started to open the way for psychodrama; Bermudez's psychodrama also became more influential, with many psychiatrists and psychologists already starting to practise it before the end of the 1960s.

Another important event at this conference was a public psychodrama session directed by Bermudez. According to Di Loreto, all those who were present at the session watched it with a mixture of horror and fascination, because from an ethical point of view the session was unacceptable. 'In half an hour he [Bermudez] exposed the internal world of the protagonist with such a degree of profundity that would take years with any other method' (Borba twelfth video 1998). Following this first public psychodrama, Bermudez directed several more sessions at the different psychiatry departments of the São Paulo hospitals, events that were talked about for weeks afterwards.

An interesting and decisive event for psychodrama happened after Bermudez's presentation at the Paulista Medical School. After the session Di Loreto had a chance to meet and have a conversation with Bermudez while he and his team were waiting for their driver to come and take them to the beach. Due to an accident, the driver did not arrive and so Di Loreto offered them a lift in his own car. When they had arrived at the beach, Bermudez invited him to stay and so Di Loreto spent three days with the team, developing a personal friendship with Bermudez (Borba twelfth video 1998).

The following year (1968) Di Loreto invited Bermudez to spend his January holidays in São Paulo, asking if he would run a 15-day psychodrama course at the Enfance Clinic, and spend another 15 days on the beach in an apartment rented for him by the clinic.

Di Loreto (together with Michael Schwarzchild) was a very successful child psychiatrist, working both at the Enfance Clinic and the psychiatry department of the São Paulo Hospital. Later on they also established a therapeutic community for children, where they used psychodrama.

When in late 1967, Di Loreto was trying to select the professionals for Bermudez's course, it was not possible for him to restrict the selection only to his colleagues from the Enfance Clinic. Many other requests arrived from various groups and institutions. With the consent of Bermudez, three separate groups were formed, each consisting of more than ten professionals (totalling 37 altogether). The work they did consisted of both psychotherapy and seminars (Borba twelfth video 1998).

Bermudez's psychodrama course

After completing this initial course, the Brazilian professionals came together for a meeting and decided to contract Bermudez and his team in order to continue the training they started, asking him if he could come and stay in São Paulo for one week every two months. A committee was formed with a representative of each institution present at this meeting: the psychiatry unit of the São Paulo Hospital, the psychiatry unit of the Clinical Hospital, National Institute of Social Providence (INPS), the Juqueri Hospital, the psychology section from the Sedes Sapientae Institute, the psychology section of the São Paulo University and the Brazilian Psychoanalytic Society from São Paulo. Out of the 37 students (who were part of the first training), the following were chosen as representatives: A.C. Cesarino, Laércio Lopes, P.P. Uzeda Moreira, J.M. D'Alessandro, Íris Soares Azevedo, A.C. Soeiro, Michael Schwarzchild and Deocleciano Alves. These professionals became the directorial board of the São Paulo Psychodrama Study Group (GEPSP), with the objective to organize Bermudez's visits to Brazil. There were a great number of professionals interested in the training and so by the end of 1968 five training groups were designated (G1, G2, G3, G4 and G5), comprising 68 students altogether (Borba third video 1993; the GEPSP Bulletin).

The training was done on two different levels: training for directors, only for doctors (with the exception of Íris Azevedo, who was a psychologist); and training for auxiliaries, both for doctors and psychologists. Students were accepted only if they were in their final year of (medical or psychology) studies. Sessions were held in five private consultation offices, where special psychodrama rooms were built and equipped for the training.

Over that year Bermudez's 68 students met for five training weeks. Within these intense training periods they were completely dedicated to psychodrama. The groups met in the morning, afternoon and evening for therapy sessions, theoretical seminars and for role-play sessions, where they could practise the roles of director, trained auxiliary and supervisor. Under the military dictatorship, this psychodrama course was like an oasis of freedom.

In February 1969, three new training groups were established (N1, N2, N3 – N standing for new) which comprised another 59 professionals. Within these groups were such well-known therapists as Eva Gaudêncio, Regina Chnaiderman, Gaiarsa, Vera França and others (GEPSP Bulletins).

Even though now it counted 128 students, the directorial board of GEPSP remained the same as it had been elected originally. Considering that these directors were elected in a democratic way, the increase in the number of students should have resulted in a new election; however, this never happened. The eleventh issue of the GEPSP Bulletin informed the readers that the study group had become affiliated to the Argentinean Psychodrama Association, in order to become part of the World Centre of Psychodrama, which had Moreno as its president. The new training groups started to practise therapy with an Argentinean psychiatrist and psychodramatist trained by Bermudez, Dr Jose Echanis. Some of the more advanced Brazilian trainees (the directors of GEPSP) also started to lead study groups and role-play sessions.

This way, even though all 37 members of the original study group were still part of the training, it was the privilege of the six directorial members only to assume the trainer function so early on. A sense of dissatisfaction developed towards the GEPSP administration: the power was concentrated exclusively in the hands of Bermudez and the directorial board. However the proximity of the Argentinean Conference and the preparation of the work that was going to be presented there, postponed the crisis to the following year.

In August 1969 the fourth International Psychodrama and Sociodrama Conference was held in Argentina with the participation of both Moreno and Zerka. At this conference Bermudez was raised into the international heights of psychodrama (Borba twelfth video 1998). He had been in contact with Moreno for six years and had become more and more involved on the international psychodrama scene. At the conference the Brazilians presented much of their work and were so successful that it was decided that the following conference, the fifth, would be held in São Paulo (even though it ought to have been in Europe).

In September 1969 a new course ('Dramatic techniques used in teaching') was introduced at the GEPSP; the course was run by Maria Alice Romaña (also Argentinean) who, as part of Bermudez's team, had been working on this topic since the beginning of the 1960s. Four new groups were formed with pedagogic orientation, for pre-elementary, elementary and secondary school teachers. The Brazilian psychotherapists D'Alessandro and Uzeda Moreira were both part of the pedagogic team. This course had become a great success and the number of students at GEPSP rose to 168 (GEPSP Bulletins; Borba fifth video 1995).

In December 1969 three more training groups for therapeutic psychodrama were established (NN1, NN2 and NN3 – NN standing for the newest). These students had psychotherapy and supervision with Dr Gaston Mazieres (from the Argentinean team), but they were also trained by the Brazilians from the directorial board of GEPSP. The numbers of students was now over 200 (GEPSP Bulletins).

The fifth International Psychodrama and Sociodrama Conference was organized in São Paulo between 16 and 22 August 1970. Before the conference an informative bulletin was published, which contained extracts of the farewell talk given by J. L. Moreno on 27 August 1969 at the fourth International Conference in Buenos Aires:

> I started to create and it is now your responsibility to continue this creation; to continue to work towards the final form of humanity and towards peace, because without creativity people will end up killing each other. I leave to you my son Rojas-Bermudez and my daughter Zerka; I also leave to you psychodrama and group dynamics. However, it is important that you don't just take this knowledge as from dead books, but try and live through this knowledge in order to find the solution. ...I believe with certainty that you should start already here, in Buenos Aires. There are many countries in Latin America: so you should organize a conference every year. This however, shouldn't be a conference of words but a conference of action, a conference that teaches you how to live. Because psychodrama is a method that teaches all of us – doctors, husbands, wives – how to live... For this reason we decided that next year's conference should be in Brazil in the city of São Paulo. Greetings to Brazil!

As it turned out later on, Moreno's words made a good advertisement for the conference in 1970. The conference was organized by GEPSP, supported by the World Centre of Psychodrama, Sociometry and Group Psychotherapy and the Argentinean Psychodrama Association, under the auspices of the Medical School of the São Paulo University.

The conference had the following themes: psychodrama and psychotherapy, sociodrama, psychopharmacology, institutional psychiatric assistance, communitarian therapy, learning and mental hygiene.

However, the climate of dissatisfaction related to the power issues around the directorate of GEPSP and the communication issues between the directorate and trainees, still persisted. Nevertheless these problems were put to one side yet again, because everybody had to dedicate themselves to the preparation of the conference that was going to be held jointly with the first International Conference of Therapeutic Communities.

The 1970 conference and the split

All the institutions, clinics and therapeutic centres were busy with work, study and the organization of the conference. In mid-1970 two new courses were introduced at GEPSP: 'Therapeutic community' and 'Psycho-dance' (GEPSP Bulletins). The Educational Secretary of São Paulo offered the São Paulo Museum of Arts as the venue for the conference.

Many other institutions also helped with the organization: the World Association of Psychiatrists, the Brazilian Association of Psychiatrists, the São Paulo Psychology Society, the Psychiatry Department of the São Paulo Medical School, the Holy House of São Paulo, the University of Campinas, the Sedes Sapientae Institute, the Moreno Institute and the Psychiatric Unit of the São Paulo Hospital.

In contrast with the unsuccessful early attempts of the psychoanalytic movement, psychodrama received academic support fairly early on. Because in São Paulo city there were more than 150 psychiatrists and psychologists who were working with psychodrama, it was not possible to exclude psychodrama from the curriculum of university and post-graduate courses.

The fifth International Psychodrama Conference was opened jointly with the first International Conference of Therapeutic Communities, on 16 August 1970, with the participation of around 3,000 people. Among the participants were: psychiatrists, psychologists, teachers, many artists, psychotherapy patients, sociologists and numerous camouflaged agents of the secret police (representing the dictatorship) (Borba, second video 1993).

It is hard to imagine how a group of professionals, with only two and a half years of training, were able to organize an event of such magnitude. At the opening of the conference the directorial members of GEPSP – being the only ones who had completed their training – were awarded the diploma of psychodrama trainers. Six of them became trainers for the whole of Brazil: Azevedo, Cesarino, Moreira, Lopes, Soerio and D'Alessandro.

Many well-known psychodramatists from all around the world also attended, representing countries such Nigeria, Switzerland, Scotland, Argentina, USA, Colombia, Spain, France, Holland and Japan. Moreno and Zerka however, were not able to attend.

Bermudez's quick rise on the scene of Latin-American psychodrama, the power struggles and the political immaturity of the GEPSP members resulted in a strong sense of dissatisfaction. Pundik, an Argentinean psychodramatist closely connected to Moreno, left the conference and went to Beacon. He returned bringing messages of dissatisfaction from Moreno. Bermudez was strongly criticized for his multiple roles within the training of the G groups (therapist, supervisor, and trainer) and now also being one of the organizers and the honorary vice-president of the fifth International Conference.

After the event, the eleven groups training in therapeutic psychodrama set up a meeting of their representatives. The so-called Group of Eleven was formed, consisting of a representative chosen from each of these groups. They composed and sent a letter to the directorial board of GEPSP, in which they complained about the lack of communication between the directorate and the associates of the GEPSP and the lack of participation of the associates in the decision making. They also stated that they no longer considered the directorial board of GEPSP as being representative of the training organization.

They suggested the formation of a provisory committee consisting of the eleven representatives already elected by the training groups. They also demanded that the actual members of the directorate should not be allowed to become candidates for the new directorial board. And finally, they proposed the elaboration of a statute before February 1971. In their letter they also made it clear that they had no intention of boycotting the course, on the contrary, they wanted GEPSP to become a democratic institution.

When receiving the committee of the eleven representatives, in response to their demands Bermudez stated that they were 'making a revolution of the poor', characteristic of the underdeveloped countries of Latin America.

Of the 142 associates of GEPSP, 113 signed a petition in which they stated that the Group of the Eleven were representing their interests. They also demanded from the directorate (that had already been in power for two years and eight months) a financial report of this period and a clarification of the existing relationship between GEPSP and the Argentinean Psychodrama Association. The petition also demanded the creation of a statute for a new society. They wanted these demands to be approved by an assembly that would also be the cradle of the São Paulo Psychodrama Society. What the students really wanted was a Brazilian society independent of the Argentinean Psychodrama Association.

The petition was signed on 8 October 1970, and the students stated that they would only return to their training activities after their demands were met. This document led to the splitting of GEPSP. In a meeting held on 9 October 1970, Laercio Lopes, Antonio Cesarino and Uzeda Moreira announced the split to the other directorate members and Bermudez. On 30 October a letter arrived from Moreno in which he communicated that the Argentinean Psychodrama Association was no longer a member of the World Centre of Psychodrama. This represented the end of the São Paulo Psychodrama Study Group.

Between October and December 1970 the two subgroups that survived the extinction of GEPSP met and prepared the statute for the foundation of their own separate societies. Marisa Greeb came to one of the meetings of the Group of Eleven, asking to become a member of the society as a representative of pedagogical psychodrama. The group told her that she could become an associate but would have no right to vote, because the institution was formed only for psychotherapists. Greeb, together with Maria Alicia Romaña founded a Role-Playing Institution in 1971 (Borba sixth video 1995).

In December 1970 the Brazilian Psychodrama and Sociodrama Association (ABPS) was founded, having as trainers Íris Soares Azevedo, J.M. D'Alessandro and A.C. Soeiro. The São Paulo Psychodrama Society (SOPSP) was also founded, having as its trainers A.C. Cesarino, Laércio Lopes and Uzeda Moreira.

In this way, psychodrama was definitely established in Brazil. Within the first few years of the 1970s these two institutes, together with the ones that were set up by Pierre Weil, gave birth to another 14 therapeutic psychodrama institutions, which in 1976 – thanks to the efforts of many psychodramatists led by José Fonseca – founded the Brazilian Psychodrama Federation (FEBRAP), whose first president was Içami Tiba.

Notes

1 Originally published under the title: 'A chegada do psicodrama no Brasil – sua história de 1960 a 1970'. *Revista Brasileira de Psicodrama 9*, 2, pp.11–36, 2001.
2 This project resulted in a series of video recorded interviews with the pioneers of Brazilian psychodramatists, see below.
3 Otto Kleinberg was an American social psychologist at the Columbia University, who was familar with sociometry and psychodrama.
4 The following is a list of video recorded interviews with the pioneers of Brazilian psychodrama, which resulted from the initiative of Carlos Borba, coordinator of the Psychodrama Remembrance Project, started in 1993.

First Video (São Paulo, Brazil, 17 September 1993)
Interviewee: Íris Soares de Azevedo – psychologist
Interviewer: Annita Malufe

Second Video (São Paulo, Brazil, 18 November 1993)
Interviewee: Antonio Carlos Cesarino – psychiatrist
Interviewer: Lais Machado

Third Video (São Paulo, Brazil, 03 December 1993)
Interviewee: Alfredo Correia Soeiro – psychiatrist
Interviewer: Annita Malufe

Fourth Video (São Paulo, Brazil, 22 October 1993)
Interviewee: José Manoel D'Alessandro – psychiatrist
Interviewer: Annita Malufe

Fifth Video (São Paulo, Brazil, 07 December 1995)
Interviewee: Maria Alicia Romaña – teacher
Interviewer: Lia Fukuy

Sixth Video *I* (Brasília, Brazil, 04 August 1998)
Interviewee: Pierre Weil – psychologist
Interviewer: Marilene M. Marra

Seventh Video (London, England, 27 September 1998)
Interviewee: Anne Ancelin Schutzenberger – psychologist
Interviewer: Ronaldo Pamplona

Eighth Video (São Paulo, Brazil, 11 November 1993
Interviewee: Laercio Lopes – psychiatrist
Interviewer: Ronaldo Pamplona

Ninth Video (Porto Alegre, Brazil, 31 October 1982)
Interviewee: Eduardo Pavlovsky – psychiatrist
Interviewer: Ronaldo Pamplona

Tenth Video (São Paulo, Brazil, 1984)
Interviewee: Iris Soares de Azevedo – psychologist
Interviewers: Vivian Bonafer Ponzoni, Marta Brunier and Maria Cristina Oliveira

Eleventh Video (São Paulo, Brazil, 09 May 1994)
Interviewee: Mother Cristina Doria – psychologist, director of the Sedes Sapientae Institute
Interviewer: Annita Malufe

Twelfth Video (São Paulo, Brazil, 15 October 1998)
A discussion between Miguel P. Navarro and Oswaldo Di Loreto – psychiatrists

Thirteenth Video (São Paulo, Brazil, 31 August 1986)
Interviewee: Jaime Rojas-Bermudez – psychiatrist
Interviewer: José Fonseca and his team

2

The development of psychodrama theory in Brazil[1]

Sergio Perazzo

It is perhaps the inheritance from our Portuguese ancestors that we tend to wait for the return of kings disappeared in remote battles with Moorish names. It is a kind of 'sebastianism',[2] waiting for the impossible resurrection of a dead hero, who would save us from all our impasses and fears.

One of our other interesting characteristics is our idea of the winter. Still today we think of winter in terms of European or North-American images of snow; an image engraved into us by Christmas cards full of reindeer, chimneys and scarves. This image however, is very different from the humid and warm Amazon 'winter' and from our all-year long insistent and lush tropical green, that cannot be disturbed even by the occasional frosts of the southern areas.

As a consequence, even our climatic reality seems to have colonially adjusted to a non-Brazilian model of the changing seasons, as if technological development, per capita income, GDP and the snow would all be the same thing.

Just as the Portuguese were immobilized by their nostalgic waiting for Dom Sebastião, there is also a danger that we Brazilian psychodramatists will follow a similarly painful fate connected to Moreno's ghost; a fate that would comfort but also paralyse us.

In our 'nostalgia for the snow', we tend to turn towards the foreign contributors of psychodrama, and their ways of approaching and practising it. We shouldn't forget however, the specifically Brazilian psychodrama theory developed in a polymorphous way, that is, to look at our own 'tropical winter' with its lush green.

In other words, if we only 'wait for Moreno' to come and rescue us from our hesitations, falters and limitations, there is a risk that we will forget to value the different Brazilian contributions to psychodrama theory; that we will stop reflecting on our own practise that has proved able to produce solid, firm and important extensions to the original Morenian theory, even if it hasn't managed yet to answer all the questions resulting from our doubts.

I believe that it is important to be loyal and faithful to the basic and original Morenian ideas; this, however, doesn't mean that we also need to rigidly follow them. We also need to be flexible, and try to trace back through a critical perspective, the historical course of the Brazilian developments in the psychodrama theory and practise.

One of the greatest difficulties that, as psychodramatists, we have when discussing the relevant issues of psychodrama, is that it does not occur to us to clarify which aspect or level we talk about: the philosophical, theoretical or technical level. It was Santos (1989) who first drew our attention to this conceptual jumble, for example in connection with the concept of *encounter* (being part of the philosophy of the moment), or the concept of *tele* (a sociometric concept), and so on. Or, what is even worse is to connect the concept of tele with the concept of encounter, that is, connecting two concepts that belong to different categories of research and examination.

Thus, when talking about Moreno, it is important to clarify to which Moreno we refer: do we talk about the philosophical Moreno, the theoretical Moreno, or Moreno as the creator of an action method, using techniques derived from theatre? Just by simply differentiating between these three Morenos, we already create a perspective in which all three of these aspects have a different qualitative value and profundity.

Looking back over the last 35 years of Brazilian psychodrama, we can count approximately a hundred books and more than a thousand articles, as well as innumerable unpublished theses and monographs. In the following paragraphs I will highlight some of the most significant moments of these 35 years that will give the reader a sense of the direction in which the Brazilian psychodrama movement has developed.

The beginnings of the Brazilian psychodrama movement

The Brazilian premiere of the Morenian therapeutic theatre took place towards the end of the 1960s, and it made a strong impression through the power and results of its technique.

In the late sixties our country was going through a cultural effervescence and excitement on the one hand, and very strong political oppression on the other. It was a period when even the word 'gathering' could put people in danger of being denounced and arrested. Psychodrama, which until then was only considered in connection with the arts and creative processes (not to mention that it favoured group issues), appeared as an alternative to the elitist psychoanalysis. So, it is not surprising that psychodrama started to be regarded as the 'horn of plenty' by the psychiatrist, psychologists and educators of that era.

As a result, from very early on a great number of professionals became attracted to this pioneering movement of psychodrama training. Since among these professionals there were numerous respectable university professors, well established psychotherapists and even psychiatry and psychology service leaders, psychodrama had very rapidly gained both significance and respect in São Paulo.

For the same reason, it was not by chance that within this early period the theoretical teaching of psychodrama was strongly interconnected with the contributions of psychoanalysis, the anti-psychiatry movement, ethology and communication theory. Without doubt, this also had another, maybe not so clearly recognized function: Moreno's insufficiently systematized ideas were re-evaluated by these professionals who had a solid theoretical background and a heightened critical potential. I believe that this was the starting point of the Brazilian infidelity towards Moreno.

Rojas-Bermudez's 'nucleus of the I' theory (Rojas-Bermudez 1977) was based on Moreno's concept of the psychosomatic roles and Pichon-Riviere's (an Argentinean social psychoanalyst) theory of area integration. Both Bermudez and his theory had a strong influence in the orientation of the first Brazilian psychodramatists.

When formulating his ideas, Bermudez's intention was to create a theory of development and psychopathology that will extend and expand the implementation of the psychodramatic technique. This theory was trying to fill in an evident gap left by Moreno: through the understanding of the structure of the 'I' (connected to the concept of roles that were believed to be the tangible and manifest aspects of the I within human relationships), it was trying to create a bridge between the intra-psychic and the inter-relational. Interestingly, during that period the 'nucleus of the I' theory became more important and influential in Brazil than the original contributions of psychodrama's own creator, Moreno.[3]

In 1970 the fifth International Psychodrama Conference was organized in São Paulo. This conference was a watershed for the Brazilian psychodrama movement, raising numerous disturbing questions and issues among psychodramatists. A great number of professionals abandoned psychodrama training in 1970, while the split between those remaining gave birth to the first two psychodrama organizations from São Paulo. The Brazilian Psychodrama and Sociodrama Association (ABPS) has stayed faithful to the Bermudian tradition; the São Paulo Psychodrama Society (SOPSP) invited the Argentinean Dalmiro Bustos, and as a result of his influence, changed its theoretical and technical direction. Another result of this split was that for the next seven years, Brazilian psychodrama was focused more on its effort to continue the training of psychodramatists, than on producing scientific work.

The arrival of Dalmiro Bustos (in the mid-seventies) aroused a new critical conscience in the psychodrama movement. From the perspective of the psychodrama practise, Bustos (1974) introduced the Morenian phase of 'sharing', replacing what until then was called the 'phase of comments and analysis'. This in itself had revolutionized the psychodramatists' attitude towards their clients to its most profound foundations. Bustos also revaluated the action method, demonstrating its possible association with the concept of transference. Still today this view is often criticized by the Brazilian psychodramatists, for being inspired more by the Kleinean than the Morenian theory.

Bustos also introduced individual bi-personal psychodrama (without an auxiliary ego) and individual multi-personal psychodrama (with auxiliary ego) in Brazil. This has resulted in still ongoing discussions and debates regarding the place and role of the psychodrama theory within the one-to-one psychotherapy setting; a setting that before the arrival of Bustos was predominated only by psychoanalysis. Would psychodrama account for a theory of intra-psychic phenomenon? This is where this question originated.

Bustos (1975) characterized his own work as psychodramatic psychotherapy, which resulted in a revision of the term 'psychodrama'. Even when describing his other ideas (such as his role theory of clusters,[4] for example), Bustos (1979) considers sociometry to be the central or focal point of psychodrama theory. Thus he recovered the importance of socionomy and its different branches.

As a direct result of this new theoretical influence, a new trend appeared among the Brazilian psychodramatists: they started to question the 'nucleus of the I' theory, removing it from its central position in the psychodrama theory. Two radical sides developed, one defending, the other opposing Bermudez's theory and approach. Strong feelings and emotions – which originated in the 1970 split and were clearly slanted by personal issues – were ignited and re-ignited. This resulted (during the conferences of the following few years) in numerous unforgettable scenes of confrontation between psychodramatists, both of the intellectual and personal order.

Finally, at the 1977 psychiatry and mental hygiene conference (Curitiba), a definite direction and course was set for the Brazilian psychodrama movement. Many psychodramatists from Curitiba (trained by the pioneers from São Paulo) were among the organizers of the conference, and suggested the inclusion of psychodrama presentations and workshops into the programme.

Through the workshops, round-table discussions and presentations of this 1977 conference, psychodrama was finally resurrected and it regained its respectability. A new generation of psychodramatists was born: those who trained and qualified during the 1970s, in various cities around Brazil.[5] Beyond being the first opportunity for these psychodramatists to meet and get to know each other, the necessity had also arisen for a forum that would allow the exchange and the propagation of psychodramatic ideas; this suggestion was enthusiastically supported by the older psychodramatists. The conference was also a landmark of peaceful collaboration between psychodramatists coming from different traditions, and it played a significant role in the life of the then only recently founded Brazilian Psychodrama Federation (FEBRAP). The following year (1978) the first Brazilian Psychodrama Conference was organized together with the publication of the first psychodrama journal (*Revista da FEBRAP*; today called *Revista Brasileira de Psicodrama* [Brazilian Journal of Psychodrama]). Brazilian scientific psychodrama writings and work became alive again, and the pride of being a psychodramatist was restored.

Theoretical developments in the Brazilian psychodrama

As a result of the resurrection of Brazilian psychodrama, an explosion of Brazilian contributions to the scientific literature began.

In 1977, in a not widely known or remembered article, Souza Leite systematized both the positive aspects and the criticism of Bermudez's 'nucleus of the I' theory. It was he who first noted the similarities between the areas described by Bermudez and Pichon-Riviere; but he also criticized Bermudez for not expanding more on the subject. Souza Leite was already looking for ways to move forward from this theory, for ways to fill in the gaps in the theory.

In an unpublished monograph, Campedelli (1978) opened up the discussion and argument regarding individual bi-personal psychodrama, setting in place and justifying this practise introduced by Bustos. Later on, through the analysis of Moreno's protocol regarding the case of Mr Rath, this topic was resumed by Nabholz, Capelato, Pierozzi *et al.* (1981). I have already mentioned the conceptual implications resulting from Bustos's practise in the previous section.

Eva (1978) started to look at the differences both in the foundations and the functioning of psychodrama therapy groups and analytical therapy groups. In this respect he compelled psychodramatists to consider group processes from the perspective of the psychodramatic action, also taking into consideration the rules and laws of psychodrama in managing and dealing with the group process.

In 1979 and 1980 two important books were published that had a very significant effect on the new evolutionary direction of the Brazilian psychodrama theory; these two books are also essential in order to understand the later developments of Brazilian psychodrama. The first book was written by Alfredo Naffah Neto (1979) and was entitled: *Psychodrama: Decolonizing the Imaginary*. The author of the second book was José Fonseca (1980), and his book was entitled: *The Psychodrama of Madness – Correlations between Buber and Moreno*.

In his book, Naffah Neto suggested a profoundly critical revision of Moreno's role theory, spontaneity and creativity theory as well as his socionomic project. He also created and introduced some new and original concepts that in my view are fundamental in filling in some of the gaps in the Morenian theory. One of these was the concept of the 'imaginary roles',[6] introduced as a new role category that differs from the psychodramatic roles. Naffah Neto's redefinitions brought more clarity to those aspects of the psychodrama theory that until then were more sparse and incomplete both in their content and form. As far as I know, there were no other similar writings published in the international psychodrama literature. In my view this is Naffah Neto's most valuable contribution; I consider it even more important than his psychodrama writings written from the perspective of dialectic materialism.

As part of the Naffah Neto's attempt to create a psychopathology theory, in his book he introduces the first critical thoughts on the concept of psychosomatic roles. His starting point was the 'nucleus of I' theory, which (similarly to Bustos) he considered to be too strongly underpinned by physiological mechanisms and genetic structures. Just as Bustos did, Naffah Neto also supported the inclusion of psychiatric diagnosis, mental illness and psychopathology into psychodrama.

He described the stage of the recognition of the I and of the other as being a symbolic realm of the social being. In this book we also find the first Brazilian references to Rocheblave-Spenlé, a French sociologist who critically but also brilliantly systematized the role theory.

Between the publication of these two books, Zerka Moreno had visited Brazil and publicly stated some of her critique towards J. L. Moreno's practical work, thus approving the theoretical supplements, extensions and ways of dramatizing introduced in Brazil by Bustos.

In his book published in the following year, through expanding the developmental phases and his understanding of the matrix of identity, José Fonseca (1980) created a new development theory and a psychodramatic psychopathology. This theory has become known among the Brazilian psychodramatists as the 'matrix of identity theory'.[7]

As with many other Brazilian psychodramatists, Fonseca was also strongly dissatisfied with Bermudez's 'nucleus of the I' theory. The majority of these psychodramatists however, were not sure how to create a better systematization of Moreno's postulates – it was Fonseca who did this job.

In the same year (1980), Anibal Mezher published an article in which – based on the ideas of Rocheblave-Spenlé – he critically reviews the concept of the psychosomatic roles, proposing the substitution of the term with 'corporal zones in interaction'.[8] The importance of this article was, however, not fully recognized at that time.

The ideas introduced by Naffah Neto, Fonseca and Mezher had finally supplied the unsatisfied psychodramatists with that missing theoretical framework which they were looking for in connection with the 'nucleus of the I' theory.

As with how Bermudez's views were originally received, Fonseca's new theory also resulted in a shift in the focus of the psychodrama theory. The 'matrix of identity' theory was placed into the centre of psychodrama theory, and for some years the latter was almost completely dominated by the former. This was reflected in the great number of articles written by Brazilian psychodramatists who were treating the subject of the matrix of identity, and also in the fact that this theory was strongly emphasized in all psychodrama training courses.

Maybe it was due to this excessive preoccupation with Fonseca's theory, that in 1982 Almeida's book entitled *Open Psychotherapy: The Psychodrama Method* did not receive all the attention that it deserved. By bringing together diverse and different views regarding the psychodrama theory Almeida supported and defended the definition and classification according to which 'the psychodrama method is a comprehensive existential-phenomenological method, and for this reason it is an open psychotherapy'. Who knows, maybe we would have reflected more on Almeida's ideas, if at the time we had been allowed a better and more inclusive view that would illuminate the obscure areas of psychodrama theory, without segmenting it so radically.

The 1980s were the most productive period of scientific psychodrama writings in the history of Brazilian psychodrama, the majority of these contributions being focused on the description of technique and theoretical details.[9] In the following paragraphs I will present some of those contributions which I consider to be fundamental pillars of psychodrama theory.

I would like to mention here two significant books written in this period: the first one was entitled *The Theatre of Anarchy* and was written by Moyses Aguiar (1988); the second *Oedipus: The Psychodrama of Destiny* by João Altivir Volpe (1990). Through these books Aguiar and Volpe recovered the concept of psychodrama as 'therapeutic theatre'[10] (derived from the theatre of spontaneity, traditional theatre and the Greek theatre), emphasizing its social and cathartic power and potential. It was probably these writings that influenced Luis Falivene Alves (1990) to describe in more detail the concept of protagonist, differentiating it from the group emergent or representative.[11] These three authors redefined drama and its place, and also introduced the concept of the 'hidden plot'.

Through a profound and objective analysis Aguiar (1991) has also revised the concept of tele (previously studied by Manoel Dias Reis), giving a historical overview of Moreno's definitions and their modifications within his work, and pointing out both the strengths and omissions of his theory. He also introduced some corrections of the theory such as the current (actual), residual and virtual links, and the dramatic project, for example.

Further to this, to only mention some of his contributions, Aguiar reformulated the concepts of tele and transference.

Aguiar was the first to observe the incoherence of references regarding the matrix of identity in Moreno's work. This gave me the impulse to expand more on this topic, trying to demonstrate through an analysis of Moreno's work (backed up by Garrido-Martin), that the matrix of identity is inconsistent within the Morenian theory. Since in Moreno's book *Psychodrama* the concept of the matrix of identity has been only mentioned within a few paragraphs in the chapter on spontaniety, in my view (Perazzo 1992) this concept should not have become the main theoretical core of psychodrama. Sociometry, the role theory and the spontaneity-creativity theory on the other hand, are much more inter-connected, and so these should have a more central position in psychodrama theory.

In addition to similar thoughts regarding tele and transference, Aguiar and I also both sustain the view that in his writings Moreno did not intentionally elaborate a theory of development, personality and psychopathology that would be consistent with the inter-relational focus of psychodrama. In my understanding, the connection with the intra-psychic phenomena happens through roles that – according to Rocheblave-Spenlé – are intimately and indirectly correlated with the personality.

In one of his more recent writings (under the influence of Nietzche, Deleuze and Guattari) Naffah Neto (1990) wrote: 'in order to be defined, the psychodramatic concepts need at least two theoretical axes: a topology of the superficial (external) and a dynamic of the (internal) currents or fluxes'. By 'superficial' he means the outline or periphery of the bodies and their contacts (that is the inter-relational), while by 'flux' or 'current' he means our own being with its existential movements (the intra-psychic).

As all the above-presented theoretical approaches demonstrate, there are many different ways to investigate the relationship of the inter-relational and the intra-psychic, the relationship of the individual and the group, the relationships of the act(ion) and method. In this investigation some psychodramatists made an attempt for a critical elaboration of Moreno's psychodrama theory; another author created a 'nuclear' theory removing some of the Morenian aspects from it; others tried to fill in the gaps of the theory by using a psychoanalytic perspective; some psychodramatists abstracted the symbolic content in order to examine the relational structure through the communication theory (leaving sociometry at the side); while some others were inspired by the systemic theory widely used in contemporary Spanish and German psychodrama.[12]

We also have a tendency to discuss more general psychotherapy issues, but say almost nothing or very little about psychodrama theory itself. I think that this actually reflects our anxieties related to our everyday practise, and the sometimes solitary role characteristic of therapists, trainers or supervisors. We don't always discriminate between psychotherapy in general and psychodrama, just as what psychodramatists write doesn't always necessarily refer exclusively to the theory of psychodrama.

As Vera Cecilia Motta Pereira accurately pointed out, psychodrama used with children often doesn't go beyond being play-therapy, not very well disguised behind a mask or façade of psychodrama; this field of application tends to more use an arsenal of toys rather than the theoretical arsenal of psychodrama. I would like to mention Camilla Salles Gonçalves (1988), who has done significant psychodramatic work in this area.

Similarly, when used with adolescents, psychodrama often simply just returns to a general understanding of adolescence instead of actually creating a psychodrama theory applied to adolescence. Maria Alice Romaña (1989) made some attempts to understand and recover Moreno's ideas related to adolescence. Similarly, José Roberto Wolff (1985) has recovered Moreno's psychodramatic views regarding dreams.

Not long ago a psychodramatist asked me the following question: 'How do we work with neo-psychodrama?' – a clear reference to Fonseca's (1992) article entitled 'Psychodrama or neo-psychodrama?'. This question well reflects our anxiety to incorporate new techniques, but without examining their content. I would like to emphasize here that Fonseca created the term 'neo-psychodrama' with the intention of characterizing the present developmental phase of psychodrama, rather than describing a certain trend, current, point of view or way of practising psychodrama. It is more of a historical label, similar to the terms used to describe phases of art history, such as neo-classicism or post-modernism. Since it is not purely Morenian anymore, the Brazilian psychodrama movement can be considered to belong to this period, called 'neo-psychodrama' by Fonseca. I would also like to point out that in this present developmental phase of psychodrama there is a potential risk for the distortion of concepts; we need to remember not to assimilate without criticism all the aspects resulting from the diffusion of sociometry.

Over the last few years a tendency has developed among Brazilian psychodramatists to be critical and spiteful regarding the Morenian project. I believe that beyond being critical, it is important to try and gain a full picture of Moreno: we need to try and see his skills and wisdom as well as his mistakes and shortcomings, to see his genius and his mediocrity, his revolutionary ideas and the gaps in his psychodrama theory. However, even if his theoretical contributions have some omissions, this doesn't mean that we should minimize or undervalue their importance.

In a recent debate, Pedro Mascarenhas said, that we psychodramatists do not understand each other when we talk about the theory, and that real understanding only happens through the practise of dramatizations, where each one of us will unquestionably recognize him/herself and the others, as psychodramatists.

Taking Mascarenhas's idea further we could say that above and beyond the words and explanations, psychodrama captures and enchants by affecting and uniting us with the almost hypnotic force of its drama; a power similar to the magic of the rabbit appearing from the magician's top hat.

Just as theatre or any other form of art, psychodrama is also a reflection of the human condition (a reflection which is pale because of its limitations, but also bright and splendid because of its intensity), achieved through the means of emotions, feelings and sensations. The science only came after (the art) and changed us into psychodramatists, forgetting to call ourselves 'psycho-dramaturges', a term introduced by Aguiar.

And from this perspective, the psychodramatist or psycho-dramaturge can only be seen as a travelling artist or gipsy, a bit of an amateur actor, a bit crazy, carrying on his cart a trunk full of his own costumes made of fabric, cardboard or tin; but a trunk with its hinges stuck, awaiting to be opened and liberate the artist's dreams imprisoned by the impositions of culture; liberating them without any compromise with banality. In the absence of the means to express these dreams in paint, in a tune, in a verse, on a screen, a photo, or a mask, we need – in the marble laboratories – at least to drip them into an Erlenmeyer or a melting pot, measuring them with a simple ammeter or stirring their essence in the complex mesh of a nuclear accelerator. Certainly, this is the inevitable crossroad that psychodrama proposes for the encounter between science and art.

Notes

1. Originally published under the title: 'O desenvolvimento da teoria do psicodrama no Brasil' in S. Perazzo (1994) *Ainda e Sempre Psicodrama [Psychodrama Still and Forever]*. São Paulo: Ágora, pp.21–31.
2* Dom Sebastião was one of the last kings of Portugal (1568–1578), before the country lost its independence to Spain, in 1580. In 1578 he was on a crusade in North Africa, trying to re-conquer the Moorish territories, when on a foggy morning he disappeared in the battle of Alcacer-Quibir; a battle also symbolizing the end of the Portuguese national independence. His disappearance gave origin to a legend, that one day he might return from somewhere unknown and save the people of Portugal. Dom Sebastião, 'the Wished', the symbol of patriotism, became a mythical figure as a result of the inherent necessity of the Portuguese to create heroic figures that represent the superiority of their national values. 'Sebastianism' is the expression for this infinite and nostalgic waiting for the return of a hero, a very Portuguese feeling developed over the centuries.
3* Bermudez's 'nucleus of the I' theory is presented in Chapter 5.
4* Bustos's revision of his cluster theory is presented in Chapter 6.
5* During the seventies the pioneers of psychodrama from São Paulo started to run numerous training groups all over Brazil and thus the movement had significantly grown. José Fonseca was first invited to run training groups in Curitiba, then later on started up further training groups in Porto Alegre, Rio de Janeiro and Florianopolis. Alfredo Soeiro introduced psychodrama training in Salvador, Campinas, Ribeirao Preto, Fortaleza and Manaus, while Miguel Navarro started training groups in Goiana and Botucatu. (Fonseca 1993)
6* The concept of 'imaginary roles' introduced by Naffah Neto is discussed in detail in Chapter 7.
7* For a detailed description of this theory, see Fonseca 2004.
8* For Mezher's critical review of the psychosomatic roles, see Chapter 7.
9* In a more recent publication, Perazzo (2000) listed a great number of these contributions. It would be impossible to include the full list here, but nevertheless I would like to mention at least a few of these authors. *Geraldo Massaro* reviewed the theory of the scene and the psychodrama with psychotics; *Manoel Dias Reis* studied sociometry from a phenomenological-existential perspective; *Rosa Cukier* studied narcissism from a psychodramatic perspective; *Arthur Kaufman* and *Maria Alicia Romana* studied psychodrama from an educational and pedagogical point of view; *Albor Vives Renones* has further deepened the concept of the catharsis of integration; *Devanir Merengue* studied the relationship of psychodrama and passion, particularly the protagonist's 'out of self' state; *Anna Maria Knobel* has applied Moreno's sociometric laws to the group direction strategies; *Mariangela Pinto de Fonseca Wechsler* has correlated Moreno and Piaget as well as psychodrama and constructivism.

10* Aguiar's reflections on the therapeutic theatre are presented in Chapter 9.
11* For Falivene Alves's conceptualization of the protagonist, see Chapter 8.
12 In October 1993, in Serra Negra the first Brazilian Seminar of Psychodrama Theory was organized by the Brazilian Psychodrama Federation, representing a mature forward step in the process of structuring the psychodrama theory.

3

The roles of the colonized and the colonizer
In search of the identity of Brazilian psychodrama[1]

José Fonseca

I must admit that when invited to talk about this topic, my immediate thought was that this would be a task for social scientists. What could a psychiatrist possibly say about colonizers and the colonized? But eventually I realized that as a psychotherapist I could look at some of the psychodynamic aspects involved in the process of colonization. And since the title refers to the 'roles' of the colonizer and the colonized, as a psychodramatist I could also rely on Moreno's role theory. Moreno (1946) after all, was emphasizing the socio-cultural aspects in the development of the personality: 'The matrix of identity is the social placenta of the child.' I decided, therefore, to synthesize some of Moreno's concepts with some of my personal theoretical concepts that may be useful in discussing the roles of the colonized and the colonizer.

Moreno's role theory

Moreno describes human development from the perspective of the matrix of identity, the bio-psycho-social-cosmic cradle of the child that provides the constituents for the later development of the adult's characteristics. The matrix of identity can be understood as a relational support network; within this network the interactions with the new being are permeated by genetic, psychological and cultural aspects.

The baby's initial development in the matrix of identity happens through the psychosomatic roles. These are responsible for the child's first interactions with its environment. Within these psychosomatic roles (such as the ingestor, defecator, urinator, breather, sleeper, etc.) various biological, psychological and cultural aspects are implicitly present and mixed together. The act of suckling for example, involves the instinctive aspect of alimentation, the psychological network that surrounds the baby and also the local cultural customs related to breast-feeding. The relationship, therefore, does not depend only on one, but on two people; moreover, it doesn't depend only on two, but on many people, since the network within which the relationship happens consists of multiple influences. Thus we can say that when talking about a relationship we always refer to a group of people, that the concept of 'I alone' is a mere abstraction, and that individual psychology is basically group psychology.

In the developmental process, following the psychosomatic roles, the psychological roles appear. In order to better understand their functions, I would like to refer here to the contributions of two other psychodamatists who called these roles fantasy (Perazzo 1995) or imaginary (Naffah Neto 1995) roles. As their name also suggests, these roles are responsible for the fantasy world (conscious-unconscious). To begin with, the child cannot differentiate between fantasy and reality. This distinction or 'breach' only happens when the social roles develop. Social roles are performed in the context of social reality and in accordance with the cultural norms that are in effect within that social reality.

The role structure then, can be understood as consisting of internment psychosomatic roles, intermediary fantasy or imaginary roles and finally social roles, these latter being the apparent roles, in contraposition with the latent roles that we own. It is important to remember that both our conscious and unconscious life is involved in this process, and that roles represent the common denominator between the individual and society. In Moreno's (1946) socionomic theory 'roles are the cultural units of behaviour'. Therefore, in order to analyse the roles, we need to deal jointly with their psychological as well as social aspects. In Moreno's view the personality develops starting from the role play; in this sense psychological development represents the learning of how to play roles in life. We can also say that role play is equivalent to establishing operational relationships or connections, since a certain role can only be performed if its counter-role also exists. What would a doctor be without a patient or vice-versa? Or what would be a teacher without a student? In a spontaneous and creative relationship role reversal occurs naturally. A flowing relationship can be characterized by one's flexibility to put him/herself in the place (role) of the 'other'. In an imposed, non-democratic relationship however, role-reversal does not happen mutually. We can observe that in the spontaneous relationship of complementary roles there exists a mutual intentionality of a conscious-unconscious order. This can be observed in the act of breast-feeding for example, where both mother and child 'want' to participate in the act (these are unequal or asymmetric roles); it can also be observed in a sexual relationship, where both lovers mutually desire each other (equal or symmetric roles). In other words, there is compromise and co-responsibility (in the sense of an authentic response) in the execution of the act.

Modes and modalities of roles

In a recent writing (Fonseca 2004, Chapter 2), I suggested that through the performance of the psychosomatic and imaginary roles, different *modes* and *modalities of roles* develop that will mark (affect) the social roles and therefore will coin a certain way of being in adult life. Let us briefly overview how this happens. In the chapter I am referring to, I wrote that during the neuro-psychological development an 'internal' and an 'external' conscience is established and as a result of the movement between these two, an 'internal-external' conscience also develops. So the child learns to realize *what and how something enters him/her*, and also *what and how something exits him/her* (the recognition of the I); the child also learns *what and how he/she can place something inside the other*, and *what and how he/she can receive something from the other* (the recognition of the other). In accordance with these possibilities, two relational phases can be established in the developmental process; these are called the *incorporative-eliminatory* and *intrusive-receptive* phases. Depending on the psychological circumstances (or affective 'climate') experienced by the child, the roles that develop within these phases will have different characteristics. In a general sense we can say that the incorporative element of the incorporative-eliminatory phase is responsible (at different degrees and intensities) for the 'learning' of how to *receive–take–extort* (*rob*) and its opposite of how to *refuse–reject–repudiate* (*disgust, repugnance*). These constitute different ways (modes) of experiencing *what enters and how it enters the boundaries of the individual*. The eliminatory element of the incorporative-eliminatory phase is responsible for the 'learning' of the how to *give (emit)–project–throw (expel)* and its opposite of how to *preserve (save)–retain–capture (seize)*. These represent different ways (modes) of experiencing *what and how it exits the individual*.

Similarly, the intrusive-receptive phase, according to its way of action, leads to different role modalities. The intrusive element of this phase is responsible for the learning of how to *enter–penetrate (explore)–invade (conquer)*. It represents different ways (modes) of entering the boundaries of the other. The receptive element embodies the learning of how to *receive (accept)–defend (protect)*–conceal (*hide*). These represent different modalities of receiving the other within oneself.

The different modes and modalities of roles can be characterized by their degree and intensity, but it is also possible to study their content of activity–passivity (masculine–feminine) while being performed. The analysis of human attitudes and behaviours (as expressed in the performance of roles) can be enriched if we consider their characteristics in accordance with the relational circumstances within which these appear. In this sense the concept of health and pathology are more to do with the flexibility and adaptability of a role within a relationship (with its counter-role), than with an aprioristic analysis of its value. Depending on the relational equilibrium that exists in the studied relationship, different degrees of the same mode (for example 'enter–penetrate–invade' or 'receive–defend–conceal') can be considered adequate or inadequate. Being 'invasive' for example, is considered inadequate in case of a thief, while it is seen as adequate in case of a soldier 'penetrating' the enemy's territory. Similarly, sexually 'invading' a woman (and making her pregnant) without her consent is considered an aggressive act; but it is also considered aggressive if a woman sexually tempts a man 'concealing' her intention of becoming pregnant.

I believe that an endless number of possible interactive combinations can be opened up when looking at relationships from the perspective of these modes and modalities of roles and their relations.

The roles of the colonizer and the colonized

Now I have arrived at the more difficult part of this chapter. That is, I need to integrate the concepts presented above with the roles of the colonized and the colonizer. The first difficulty is how to apply a theory of individual psychological development to the analysis of social and political issues? The question is valid; however we should not forget that in the last century psychology (and especially psychoanalysis) many times went beyond its boundaries in order to contribute to the understanding of different areas of human knowledge. Therefore I would also like to propose that, at least as an experiment, we observe the possible correlations between the presented theoretical concepts and the roles of the colonizer and the colonized.

We saw that a harmonious relationship implies complementary roles that are performed with the criteria of mutual intentionality. Within this mutual intentionality both conscious and unconscious aspects of the process are involved. If this mutual intentionality is present, an automatic role reversal takes place and, through this role reversal the other is recognized (confirmed) as a person. The result of this act is a flow of spontaneity. There is a reciprocal acceptance that seems to involve a joyful or even sensual climate. There is an implicit 'wish' for the act to be performed. Even aggressive acts, for example those involving fighters, can have a mutual intentionality. However this does not happen in the relationship between the roles of the colonizer and the colonized. In this case there is no mutual intentionality or reciprocity; the intention is unilateral. Nevertheless, the structure of such a bond (in terms of complementary roles) still persists. From the role theory's point of view, the role of the colonizer fosters the role of the colonized, despite the fact that this latter is imposed by the former. Colonization is the result of the profile of these two roles and the way their relationship is established. This way, taking into consideration the cultural characteristics of the colonizers (whether English, French, Dutch, Spanish or Portuguese) and of the colonized (whether Brazilian Indians, descendents of the Incas, Aztecs or Africans), the result is the act of colonization. In any colonization act however, it is the colonizer who 'chooses' the colonized. Through submission and power, the colonizer does not offer, but imposes cultural and religious values. The 'truth' of the colonizer is absolute. Since, before the arrival of the colonizers, the colonized lived happily with their own gods and religions, catechesis or indoctrination can be seen as a subtle form of violence. What did the religious missionaries bring to the Latin American Indians? Did they bring peace or fear? They preached about hell and sin (among many others sexual sin), but ironically they also taught 'new' sexual positions like the one called the 'missionary position' that the Indians previously did not know. In contrast with the polygamist tendencies of the Indians, they preached monogamy (even though they did not follow it). They were promoting goodness and kindness, but often demonstrated a sadistic behaviour typical of the conquistadors.

When writing this chapter I came across the excellent book of the Brazilian sociologist José Souza Martins (1993), entitled *The Arrival of the Stranger*. In the chapter entitled 'Cannibalism and the baroque in the Latin-American culture', he makes reference to the first Brazilian historian from the seventeenth century, friar Vicente do Salvador. According to this pioneer of Brazilian history, 'in their religious fight against the lack of faith' the Portuguese loaded their cannons with Indian prisoners to fire them against the ones who resisted them. This happened more than 300 years ago to the Potiguar Indians, a tribe (living in Paraiba state of Brazil) which still to this day fights for the preservation of their roots.

I mentioned earlier on that the colonizer-conqueror-invader does not reverse roles with the colonized-conquered-invaded. Mutual intentionality is replaced with unilateral intentionality. Since the colonizer does not even recognize the value of the other (colonized), he is not interested in reversing roles. The colonized however, being obliged to recognize the invader's power, is able to do this reversal, even if in an aggressive manner. The ritual of cannibalism can be seen as a form of role reversal. The enemy is eaten and in this sense his power incorporated. The catholic invaders were horrified by this ritual, but they forgot that the sacrament of the holy communion also represents, even if only symbolically, a cannibalistic act – 'eating' the body and 'drinking' the blood of Christ. Martins (1993, p.21) mentions that in the 1960s the Parkateje Indians were badly affected by certain illnesses of the white people. Many of them died, the remaining men were occupied with hunting and there were not enough women left to look after the children. The tribal chief decided to take the children to the white people: 'You are the conquerors, and so it is your duty to raise our children.' Years later, when the tribe recovered they wanted their children, whom by this time had grown up, to be returned. According to Martins, there are many touching stories of these youngsters who only then found out that they were Indians. The majority returned.

From the perspective of the different *role modes* and *modalities*, characteristic of the *incorporative-eliminatory* and *intrusive-receptive* phases, we can analyse the topics of *what and how something enters me* and *what and how can (or can't) I receive inside me something that belongs to the other*. In terms of the original (primary) colonization we can say that the role of the colonizer can be described through the characteristics of *enter–penetrate (explore)–invade (conquer)*, while the role of the colonized through the characteristics of *refuse–reject–repudiate*. Even though I obviously identify with the colonized, I also need to recognize that a colonizer, who does not penetrate– invade–conquer, cannot really be called a colonizer. There were probably better and worse among the colonizers, however I believe that the results of colonization – in terms of the presented theory – depend not only on one or the other of the involved roles, but on their established relationship.

Under the influence of these ideas we also need to think about the long-term effects of colonization. The natural role reversal accomplished by the colonized continued and renewed itself over the years and centuries, resulting in the internalization or *incorporation* of the role of the colonizer. As a result however, the colonized reaches a double identity, possessing many characteristics of the colonizer (language, etc.). The colonized becomes confused in this ambiguity, not knowing any longer if he is the colonized or the colonizer, or both at the same time. In an extreme form of this confusion, he wishes to be equal (alike) with the colonizer. The characteristics of the colonizer come to represent a narcissistic ideal for the colonized that he wants to reach. And, at times, a peculiar attempt is made to repeat the cycle: the colonized aspires to become the colonizer and to have his own colonized people! This is perhaps the worst among the mutilations that result from the conquest. Taking into consideration that the roles of the colonizer and the colonized can be the base or anchor for other social roles, we can imagine how their characteristics will also affect other situations, as for example the male–female, employer–employee, father–son, etc. relationships. In one of the Peruvian regions, in an attempt for agricultural reform, the peasants who previously worked for the landowners, organized themselves in cooperative associations. But after a while some leaders of these associations became corrupt and started to show some of the characteristics of their formal landowners. They 'ascended' to the condition of their oppressors. Another example from Martins (1993, p.23) refers to a young peasant, who on a long bus journey was wearing Ray-Ban sunglasses. The youngster often took his glasses off in order to clean the lenses, taking very good care not to damage the golden label with the logo on it. Martins concludes: 'He did not wear the glasses in order to see, but to be seen.'

So we, the colonized of Latin-America, suffer from this ambiguity syndrome of double identity. We are colonized and in the same time wish to be colonizers, colonizers of ourselves or colonizers among ourselves. Martins (1993, p.20) says that still to this day we suffer from a ritual, cultural cannibalism that is responsible for the tradition of assimilating the other, incorporating his culture and manners. Everybody knows Macunaima, from Mario de

Andrade's book,[2] our 'hero without character', cannibalistic, 'the perfect synthesis of the Brazilian national character'. After the victory of their glorious revolution, the Mexican peasants entered Mexico City in a village procession. They were carrying the flag of the Virgin of Guadalupe,[3] but were begging for a piece of bread. 'They were the winners, but they did not know it, or did not know themselves!' (Martins 1993, p.23). When Che Guevara was killed in the Bolivian jungle, a group of poor peasants were shouting: 'Assassin, assassin!' However, when they got closer to the body, one of the peasants exclaimed: 'How young and beautiful he was!' (Martins 1993, p.23).

These are signs of dependency and subordination, the colonized identifying himself as inferior. He feels ashamed and tries to disguise his evident fragility. But someone who is hiding is afraid; afraid of being discovered. The colonized fears the critical look of the other–foreigner, whom he identifies as superior. This is an 'unequal regard' of the other, guided by symbolic values of nationality, as Vitale (1994, p.125) refers to it when writing about the shame of being Brazilian. Octavio Paz, a great Mexican thinker recalls that once when entering his house, from the threshold he asked if there was anyone inside. From inside the Indian servant responded: 'No, there is *nobody* in here!'

As colonized we internalized the other (the colonizer), but without reconstructing ourselves. We are us (ourselves) but our own enemy at the same time. We are a confusion of identities. Martins (1993) calls this contradiction the Latin-American baroque, a mixture of both tragic and comical. But this tragicomedy reveals the outlines of an identity. We evolve and regress in accordance with the different historical influences, succumbing here and there to a new, secondary colonization. The black Americans for example, have given up their strategy of trying to seem white (as they did in the 1940s and 1950s by straightening their hair) for now assuming ostensibly their African origin. Their question of identity however is still not solved, because they are not white North-Americans, but they are not Africans either. As they say, they are Afro-Americans, but they also carry a burden of an internal duplicity: on the one hand they are North-Americans and colonizers, while on the other hand colonized Africans.

In search of the identity of Brazilian psychodrama

As already mentioned above, it is important to make a distinction between primary and secondary colonization. Primary colonization refers to the original conquest. By secondary colonization I mean all the processes that happened afterwards, which, even if covert, have similar structural characteristics to primary colonization. We saw that primary colonization is a matter of power where the colonized does not have a choice. This, however, is not always true in the case of secondary colonization; in spite of the colonizer's evident pressure, in secondary colonization co-responsibility also exists. While the colonizer *enters–penetrates–exploits–invades–conquers*, the colonized *receives (accepts)–defends (protects)–conceals (hides)*. If, in secondary colonization, there is a sadistic component in the role of the colonizer, than there is also certainly a masochistic component in the role of the colonized; the colonized finds a certain pleasure in being colonized. He is ambivalent: he hates his conqueror, but at the same time also loves and imitates him; at times the colonizer even becomes the ideal that the colonized is foolishly trying to reach. The colonized resigns himself to accepting the situation. There are no victims in this situation. Enough of 'being a victim'! This is the diagnosis of our intellectual situation as colonized. We live in an internal contradiction and we need to take responsibility for ourselves. In the Dom Pedro II College (Rio de Janeiro) the geography of the city of Paris was taught up until the beginning of the twentieth century! And it wasn't the French who obliged us to do so. In order to find our true Brazilian identity, we need to develop a national socio-therapeutic technique, a national sociodrama.

The process of secondary colonization can be observed in all areas, including economy, politics, art and science. It also happens in those areas of science in which we are competent: in psychiatry, in psychology, in psychotherapy and in psychodrama. Let us now look at some aspects of this identity confusion characteristic to this area. In the past, Brazilian psychiatry had various influences, German and French psychiatry being the most significant ones. Nowadays it suffers from the prevailing influence of American psychiatry. A great number of our young psychiatrists, especially those engaged in an academic career, spend some time in the United States. They return not only with new scientific knowledge, but also with peripheral habits that have nothing to do with our culture. For example, they use a tie and a smock with pens of various colours sticking out from their top pocket. This is a uniform that gives *status*, and indicates that the individual has studied or wants to study in the United States. It is a fashion (custom) that besides having hardly anything to do with our tropical and subtropical climate, also denies the long fight that the previous generations of our doctors fought, to break free from the European dress code. In his role theory, Moreno describes different degrees of spontaneity when talking about performing roles: *role-taking* means the mere assumption or adoption of a role, including therefore the learning of the role; *role-playing* means representing and fully performing a role; and finally *role-creating* which is the possibility of creating, inventing a new role (also practising it). Copying and imitating models that belong to others are part of the learning process; the student would like to become ('grow') like his/her teacher. However, it is also part of the role practise to improve, to exchange information, to continue to grow. And creativity is very important in this growing process, because it presupposes a daring and challenging attitude, in order to surpass the 'cultural conserves', to create new models. For a few years I simultaneously trained psychodramatists in various Brazilian cities. In order to facilitate my travelling around the country, I made the training into eight hours per month, working with a different group (in a different location) every Saturday. Once one of my students came and proudly told me that he had set up his first therapy group. I congratulated him and also asked which day of the week he runs the group. To my surprise he answered: 'I run the group once a month the whole Saturday!' It did not occur to him that groups can be run on other days of the week and with shorter weekly sessions.

Not long ago I attended a public psychodrama session in the United States, where an American director was working with an American protagonist. The psychodrama I witnessed was so dramatic, so grandiloquent and had such a spirit of salvation around it, that I couldn't stop thinking about the religious missionaries. Nevertheless, the dramatization was flowing, director and protagonist understood each other and the outcome was positive. But I was left asking myself how the same psychodrama (working with the same theme) would develop with a Brazilian director and protagonist? It would be different. Not better and not worse, but very different, because our culture is different, and we live and express our feelings differently. It would be ridiculous for a Brazilian director to try and direct in the manner of an American director, or vice-versa.

The beginning of Brazilian psychodrama is linked to foreigners. Both in the states of Rio de Janeiro and Minas Gerais, psychodrama was introduced by the French Pierre Weil. In São Paulo state the two influential figures who introduced psychodrama were Jaime G. Rojas-Bermudez and Dalmiro M. Bustos, both Argentineans (Rojas-Bermudez was born in Colombia, but had his academic training in Buenos Aires). From these cradles, psychodrama spread to the other regions of the country by the means of Brazilians, so we also experienced being colonizers. Any study focusing on the origins of the Brazilian psychodrama history can bring valuable contributions on the theme of the roles of the colonizer and the colonized. Certainly, there is no Brazilian psychodramatist who is exempt from the tele-transferencial system involved in this process (our therapists were our 'colonizers'); but I believe that even transference can be creative at times. However, within this chapter, I did not intend to write about the history of Brazilian psychodrama. My objective was to look at the Brazilian (and also Latin-American) tendency of assuming the role of the colonized. I would also like to stress here, that in spite of the universal premises of the psychodrama theory, the practise of psychodrama is proposed to be permeated by the socio-cultural context of the place where it takes place. This implies the use of a relational perspective when looking at the relationship of the 'colonized' with their equals and with their 'colonizers'.

I would also like to stress the responsibility of the colonized in the process of 'secondary colonization'. As I mentioned before, this process of secondary colonization can be observed in all social and professional areas, and therefore it is our duty to take care of the identity of Brazilian psychodrama in its phase of development (and also our own development). It is our challenge to delineate the profile of the Brazilian psychodrama practise and to contribute to the contemporary Brazilian psychodrama theory.

When thinking of the Argentinean model of Brazilian psychodrama,[4] the first thought that occurs to me is that, in spite of the geographical proximity and cultural similarities of the two countries, there are also numerous differences between them. It is enough for example, to consider the music of these two countries in order to see these differences. Both tango and samba are beautiful, but completely different, as much in their movement, as in their melody and content of lyrics. I am not going to bore the reader by proving these differences, because they are obvious. The same applies to the American and French models of psychodrama. I would like to stress the importance of the fact, that as with Brazilian music, an authentic Brazilian psychodrama also exists; but it is lacking and so would need a 'tropical movement' that does not deny the foreign influences, but transforms them. This aspiration however, also brings some doubts: considering the way it is practised and viewed by its leaders, can we state that a Brazilian psychodrama already exists? At the thirteenth International Group Psychotherapy Conference (1998, London) four Brazilians (Ana Maria Knobel, Rosa Cukier, Maria Seixas and myself) presented on four consecutive days a series of workshops entitled 'The Brazilian connection'. Many foreigners attended and obviously appreciated Brazilian psychodrama. Perhaps this is an indication that our psychodrama identity has started to arise. And finally, one last question: was the influence of our colonizers already absorbed and integrated? I have more doubts than certainties about this question, but I feel it is time to reflect more on this topic. I would like to invite and encourage my Brazilian psychodramatist colleagues to become my doubles and to elaborate more on what I have only started to sketch within this chapter.

Notes

1 The original title: 'Os papéis de colonizado e colonizador: por uma identidade do psicodrama Brasileiro'. In J. Fonseca (2000) *Psicoterapia da Relação [Relationship Psychotherapy]*. São Paulo: Ágora, pp.203–216.
2* Mario de Andrade was a crucial figure of the Brazilian literary movement trying to break away from the European influences and create original Brazilian literature. His book entitled 'Macunaima' is considered one of the most important literary compositions in the Brazilian literature of the twentieth century. Macunaima, the central figure of this book, is an archetypal and symbolic image representing the traditional Brazilian Indian and black cultures. He is called the 'hero without character' because he has no individual character of his own, but represents all the different elements of the national Brazilian character; through his stories the myths and legends of the Indian and black Brazilian cultures are re-told.
3* The Virgin of Guadalupe is considered the Mother of the Americas. In 1531, on a mountain North-East from Mexico City a 'heavenly lady' appeared to a poor Tepeyac Indian, calling herself the Mother of the True God. She left her image imprinted on the Indian's 'Tilma' (a cheap fabric made of cactus plants), an image that after 465 years had still not worn away (even scientists cannot find an explanation for this!). At the place where this miracle happened, a sanctuary was built, which is today the second most frequented church in the whole world after the Vatican.
4 It is called the 'Argentinean model of Brazilian psychodrama' due to the contribution of the numerous Argentinean professionals who were invited to run psychodrama courses and seminars over the last 30 years; their influence transcends the original influence of Rojas-Bermudez and Bustos.

The role of the colonizer and the colonized
In search of the identity of Brazilian psychodrama[1]

Geraldo Massaro

I must admit that initially I felt slightly confused when trying to think about the central issues involved in this interesting topic. As colonized, how do we perceive and think about ourselves, and how can we reach an identity as Brazilian psychodramatists? Even if I think that reaching this identity is nearly impossible, I believe that discussions around this topic are fundamental in the search of our role as psychodramatists.

In order to facilitate the discussion of these issues, I decided to divide the topic into three sub-sections:

1. Where should I place the arms of my compasses in the attempt to trace the occupant and the occupied?
2. Who are the occupant and the occupied?
3. How did psychodrama, as a cultural product, adapt to the Brazilian environment?

Where should I place the arms of my compasses in the attempt to trace the occupant and the occupied?

We could place the needle of these symbolic compasses somewhere in the North and make a mark with the pencil-tip down here, below the Equator, where sin didn't exist.[2] Or should we place the needle in Argentina and the pencil-tip in Brazil? Or would it be better to locate São Paulo with the needle and scribble over the rest of Brazil with the pencil-tip? But we can also point with the needle at the social elite (attributed with the role of guardian or protector), the pencil-tip marking the people, the supposedly guarded and protected. Taking into consideration the specific characteristics of our history, these thoughts will inevitably lead to the roles of the colonizer and the colonized, and so any of the above possibilities can be seen as equally valid.

In comparison to other colonized regions of the world, Latin America was occupied through a different process. Since they had no interest in the native inhabitants of Latin America, the conquistadors exterminated or eliminated them. In this sense, a new occupant was created; an occupant coming from the outside. These new occupants were an extension of their European roots. Since as a result of the colonization there were hardly any native subjects left, the occupants became subjects for themselves (occupied). The result is an only half accomplished journey: we are neither Europeans, nor Americans; we are neither colonizer, nor colonized.

This is a land where everything is foreign and nothing is foreign. We live halfway between not being and being someone else (other). Both, the fabric of our cultural constitution as well as our cultural products are coming from outside of Brazil. Our institutions, our political models, our ways of relationships and even our historical facts (with a few exceptions) originate somewhere outside. However, in our collective imagination we start to gain ownership over such products. We are Brazilian exiles in Brazil; we are exiles in our own country.

These products that originate outside are only available to a small stratum of the population, to those who have the power to buy. We could say therefore, that the true occupant consists of our economic elite. This economic elite has the illusion of being the extension of the bourgeoisie of the mother country, and is characterized by an identity that is more interested in the consumption than the creation of cultural products. Under these circumstances, the elite is trying to control the anxiety resulting form an enormous social inequality, the inheritance of a society based on slavery. I believe that in order to achieve a real identity and independence, we will need to free ourselves from the characteristics of this image of being an extension of our European roots.

Being a nation of different origins and consequently of mixed blood, we don't have a sense of pride and identity of our race. We have not developed the symbolic urge that allows every single one of us to be Brazilian in the same way as a Dutch person is Dutch, or a North-American person is North-American. The result is a reduced social organization and cohesion leading to a looseness or laxity of our cultural, political and social structures.

Our response – almost a defence – to this situation is the development of individualism. Our ethic is strongly and profoundly family based, with a strong emotive and affective character. Our sense of solidarity is restricted to this immediate domestic environment, and is unreliable in the collective sense. This fact also explains our propensity for liberal[3] professions. Every individual is trying to assert himself only for himself, generally by overvaluing the intellectual activities to the disadvantage of physical work. The underlying conflicts are hidden behind a mask or façade of superficial cordiality and religiosity and so remain unresolved. This individualism is also characteristic of our social, cultural and political structures.

Who are the occupant and the occupied?

First of all I need to clarify that in Brazil, both the occupant and the occupied are subjective and relative concepts.

We saw that the issue of the occupant and the occupied involves two different forms of interest, two different codes of ethics in an eternal conflict; we also saw that every person establishes himself according to the role he/she plays within this conflict.

The occupant comes to impose his language, his rules and his laws. He comes in order to demonstrate and to exercise his power. He is not interested in designating or appointing the land, he only wants to own it. The occupied in this sense, is just an extension of this land, and therefore also a possession of the occupant. Brazil is just the means for acquiring wealth; it can be captured easily, without any hard work. Because its economic ideology is based on individualism and the idea of trade, everything can be sold, bought or exchanged. In this respect, the occupant determines and ascertains both our structures and historical facts.

The occupied on the other hand, has been subjected in the occupant's search for land. In the absence of a more clearly delineated model, norm or identity that they could follow, the occupied acted through mimicry (copying the occupant). And so the products created by the occupied had the same characteristics as the products previously brought or imported from outside. This pleased the other (the occupant), however it resulted in the fact that Brazilians did not (and still don't) have confidence in the value of their own cultural products; they only consider these cultural products valuable, if approved by others from outside (that is, foreigners).

The occupants exercise less pressure on the more disfavoured and disadvantaged social classes, because these don't have the power to buy. It is the middle class – occupied and occupant – that receives and welcomes the cultural products that originate outside. This is also true for the cultural product of psychodrama.

How did psychodrama, as a cultural product, adapt to the Brazilian environment?

Similarly to all other cultural products, psychodrama in Brazil also emerged through ideas and customs that were pre-fabricated somewhere outside of Brazil. Moreno, the creator of psychodrama – revolutionary in his ideas – also developed his method on foreign soil (in America). Therefore, psychodrama was marked by characteristics and issues that don't belong to us Brazilians: such as its dispute with psychoanalysis, sociometry as the solution for the conflict of the world, and the 'American way of life'. Further to this, psychodrama arrived in Brazil, with the mediation of Argentinean psychodramatists, filtered through their practise.

It also arrived in an era of social transformation. This era was characterized by the world-wide counter-culture and anti-psychiatry movement. In Brazil, Brazilian theatre and cinema had just started to develop, but was soon followed by the contracting of numerous foreign screenwriters, set designers, and stage managers, a process that lasted from 1950 to 1966.

Psychodrama and psychodramatists appeared on this background, characterized by counter-culture (the questioning of well established cultural, political and social values) on the one hand and a military regime on the other. They were children of many different parents, and at the same time, children without parents.

From the beginnings we (psychodramatists) were trying to find an appropriate response to this specific situation; we were searching for an identity. We were trying to delineate our own profile as we wanted it to be. In this search however, we still haven't found all the responses.

Even though our institutions were wise and had significant knowledge, they took power for granted, as an internal condition of their functioning. Power, in its concrete form, is exercised in an ideological framework, defined by visible concrete and material forms or bodies that give structure (such as FEBRAP, the Brazilian Psychodrama Federation) and by precisely and formally articulated and stated rules and regulations (such as the different statutes of our organizations). It would be interesting to find the differences between these various statutes, as well as the ways they are managed; however, my intention is only to delineate the way the above-mentioned ideological framework functions.

The first animating force behind the development of the Brazilian psychodrama movement emerged from the breach in the child–parent relationship. As a result of this breach, the child (Brazilian psychodrama) aspired to become a parent himself (to become independent); a legitimate outcome of a great effort. After the initial chaos, this force or effort produced (created) a new object; in terms of Brazilian psychodrama this new object was the Brazilian Psychodrama Federation. On the one hand, this force was positive and systematizing; it aimed to develop an administrative structure as well as rules and regulations that would allow a good functioning of the psychodrama movement. However, under this apparently homogeneous structure, a set of less positive characteristics was also hidden. This force was conservative and believed blindly in its principles; as a result it tried to resist change. It became too entangled in administration and bureaucracy and so it forgot about its original aim, that is, the development of a Brazilian psychodrama movement. From being positive and systematizing, it became conservative and rigid, and so it led to the appearance of a second animating force.

The second animating force came from the realization, that beyond the structure, there was a need for something more, for the expansion of psychodrama. This second force aimed to transform psychodrama, to open up discussions and polemic within the movement, and thus help psychodrama evolve. The main instrument of this force was the Morenian idea that psychodrama practise should adapt to and be permeated by the social, political and cultural context of the place or country where it is applied. Through this Morenian idea it wanted to challenge and to create tension in the structures already existing. However, this revolutionary movement started to represent more individual interests, or the interests of small groups, and so it lost its role of representing the collective (the whole psychodrama movement). In its attempt to develop the identity of a more independent Brazilian psychodrama movement (to 'replace the father'), this movement changed from being honest and revolutionary, into being commanding.

Left and right; forces that create tension, and forces that are conservative: our psychodrama was led by such forces. At certain times these forces alternated, at other moments they were united in a synthesis, trying to allow reciprocity, a restructuring of the course of psychodrama. But the power in itself is not enough to develop our own identity.

So, beyond the forces involved in the internal power structure of the psychodrama movement, other forces also appeared with the mission of the instrumental use of psychodrama for the Brazilian people.

As one of the results of these instrumental efforts, psychodrama 'went out into the street'. With its passion and chances for the unexpected, the street opens up a whole different area and so it presupposes a different approach. From a social point of view, people act differently on the street. The street has a different (social) hierarchy, which is more hidden and more difficult to decipher. Relationships imply different kinds of choices and the barriers between positions and statuses become temporarily suspended. These relationships are based on a more real and concrete social practise; in their search for the denied social reciprocity and equality, specific values and ideologies are acted out (staged) within these relationships. When doing psychodrama on the street, the focus is not so much on the history of the individual, but on the individual in the history.

It is clear that psychodrama's power of social transformation will depend on how the director approaches the facts of his times. Will he help enact and stage the voice of the quiet figurants (that is, people who are always in the background)? Is he going to reveal the social experiences of the less organized social groups, helping them to take care of their destiny? Will he transform this limited space into a space of performance? Will he step beyond the individual and individualist level and reach the collective? Will he bring to the surface and question the established and 'crystallized' social structures? Will he reduce and diminish the barriers separating the different social classes? Will he, at least, create a space for social encounter?

Another instrumental use of psychodrama is represented by the open sessions held at different private clinics. Despite their richness and numerous other positive aspects, these sessions usually end up serving the training of psychodramatists. Another form of use of psychodrama are the sessions held at different institutions working with issues such as violence, AIDS, abandoned street children and other social problems.

In my view, these forms of action are the closest to the real identity of Brazilian psychodrama. Even though there are still only a few, these initiatives serve a very important and special role, and so are warmly welcomed. But we shouldn't forget that the intention is to use the instruments of psychodrama for the people themselves; it should be an instrument not using, but serving people. In this respect I would like to point out that there is an important difference between a cultural product with popular content, and a production made by the people for the people.

Another important movement in the Brazilian psychodrama (that has become stronger recently) is the search for cultural differences between our psychodrama and the psychodrama of other countries. The Ibero-American conferences represent a very valuable forum for this search of identity and cultural differences. Delineating the similarities and dissimilarities between the psychodrama of different regions and countries is very welcomed and helpful in the search of our own identity. One of the risks here is to just simply follow the way psychodrama is practised in other cultures; this would be potentially limiting for the Brazilian psychodrama. However, considering the actual stage of maturity of our psychodrama, I think this risk is very small. I've heard arguments that such intercultural and international encounters would increase our power of influence towards the outside. I would also like to make a reminder, however, that the issue is not to increase our power of influence towards the outside, but to decrease the power of external influences here in Brazil. I believe that only seeking what is outside results in superficiality and the risk of obstructing the independence for which we are striving.

Before finishing this brief description of the different ideological positions, I would also like to mention the autonomous institutions that are not affiliated to the Brazilian Psychodrama Federation, and which have been trying to create different ways of teaching psychodramatic knowledge. They play a very important role in setting contrast to and creating tension within our structures. Unfortunately though, some of these institutions are based on a disturbing individualism. Nevertheless, even if sometimes inconvenient, they still play a positive role.

This is how psychodrama works in Brazil. Its governing ideologies sometimes alternate, at other times argue and fight with each other, while at other times they are integrated. The contradictions of their practise at times remain hidden, and at other times are brought to the surface. From the perspective of psychodrama as an instrument, we need to carry on improving it by developing new techniques.[4]

None of this, however, gives a full identity to Brazilian psychodrama. The full development of this identity will only be possible when psychodrama becomes the instrument of the many (people), being available for the significant majority of the population, or in other words, when it becomes part of everyday life.

Some people argue that psychodrama would become mediocre if brought down to the level of everyday life. I, however, consider mediocre those who think that maintaining these (social) differences is necessary. And this is my main worry. If in the search for Brazilian psychodrama's identity, we only reproduce the old fashioned and rigid characteristics of the occupant, will we not only nationalize this profession?

Notes

1   Originally published under the title: 'O papel do colonizador e do colonizado: por uma identidade do psicodrama no Brasil'. *Revista Brasileira de Psicodrama* 7, 2, pp.47–52, 1999.

2* This is a reference to the romantic idea of the first colonizers who, arriving on the American continent, believed that it was a paradise on Earth, a place where sin did not exist.

3* The term 'liberal' is used within this context to mean: 'relating to or having policies or views advocating individual freedom', and so it refers to the idea of individualism.

4* Some of these new techniques developed by Brazilian psychodramatists will be presented in Part 3 of this book.

Part 2

Theoretical innovations in Brazilian psychodrama

There are many Brazilian psychodramatists who have attended to Moreno's appeal not to take his work as complete and finished. Within the past few decades professionals have made great efforts to further develop the Morenian theory, producing numerous contributions especially regarding role concept and theory. Part 2 contains some of the most significant writings by Brazilian authors concerning theoretical issues.

The first chapter of this section introduces the 'nucleus of the I' theory formulated by Rojas-Bermudez, one of the most influential professionals in the Brazilian psychodrama movement. The chapter comprehensively summarizes the various aspects of this theory: Bermudez's attempt to merge psychodramatic, psychoanalytic and physiological concepts; the concept of the 'nucleus of the I' and its relation to the psychosomatic roles; Bermudez's views on role development and physio-psychopathology; as well as the concepts of role complementarity and that of the intermediary object.

Dalmiro Bustos further elaborates on his cluster theory, analysing in depth the various dynamics involved within the different role clusters.

In a theoretical digression around the role concept, Sergio Perazzo makes an attempt to find the common denominators for the role theories of Rocheblave-Spenlé, Aníbal Mezher and Alfredo Naffah Neto. Through an in-depth analysis of the various role concepts and by introducing such terms as the imaginary role, the fantasy role, the fantastic role and the dramatic role, he aims to arrive at a more precise definition of the psychodramatic role.

Luís Falivene Alves draws our attention to the necessity for a more precise conceptualization of the protagonist as an instrument of psychodrama. Using Greek tragedy as an analogy, as well as clinical examples, he attempts to define the protagonist more appropriately, distinguishing it from the group representative (an emergent, chosen or designated group member). The author also correlates the 'protagonic theme' to the group context, and the emergence of the real protagonist to the dramatic context.

Based on the concepts of the dramatic project and focus, Moysés Aguiar describes various approaches within the psychodrama practise (such as diagnostic psychodrama, gestalt psychodrama, reparatory psychodrama, pragmatic psychodrama and the theatre of spontaneity). He discusses the therapeutic potential of the spontaneous theatre, seen as the operational model for psychodrama, sociodrama and axiodrama. Emphasizing the importance of dramatic action and co-creation, Aguiar also examines how the theatre of spontaneity can enrich the practise of psychodrama.

5

The 'nucleus of the I' theory of Jaime Rojas-Bermudez

Zoltán Figusch

Within this chapter I present the 'nucleus of the I' theory formulated by Jaime Rojas-Bermudez. This theory represents one of the most central influences within Brazilian psychodrama, while Rojas-Bermudez was one of the most influential figures in the Brazilian psychodrama movement. He has written extensively about the 'nucleus of the I' theory (Rojas-Bermudez 1977, 1978, 1984, 1985, 1997); however, translating all this work would result in a separate book in itself. Therefore, after extensive research on this topic, I eventually decided to sum up the most relevant aspects of Bermudez's theory. In the following chapter I will present the definition of the 'nucleus of the I' concept, and will also introduce Bermudez's role development and psychopathology theories which he formulated based on this concept. However, since the 'nucleus of the I' theory has its origins in Moreno's concepts regarding roles, first I will briefly review the Morenian role theory.

Moreno's role theory

In his writings, Moreno never actually used the term 'nucleus of the I'. Moreno's starting points in his great preoccupation with psychological development were the concept of the matrix of identity and role theory. Since he always looked at man (and also the infant) immersed in his social context, Moreno's role concept presupposes interrelation, interaction and action, these social aspects being crucial in the development of the roles and the self.

According to Moreno (1934, p.76), 'role emergence is prior to the emergence of the self. Roles do not emerge from the self, but the self emerges from the roles.' He considered the roles to be the embryos or forerunners of the self, and distinguished between physiological or psychosomatic roles (for example, the role of the eater, the sleeper and the sexual role); psychological or psychodramatic roles (ghosts, fairies and hallucinated roles); and social roles (parent, policemen, doctor, etc.). Thus, in his definition, the self is the totality of roles a person plays in his life, and so the development of the self is linked to the development of roles.

At the basis of this developmental process is the 'matrix of identity' (social placenta), considered by Moreno to be the 'locus' (foundation, or blueprint) from where the self and its ramifications (the roles) emerge in gradual phases. The world of the matrix of identity is an undifferentiated universe, within which the first roles to emerge are the physiological or psychosomatic roles. According to Moreno (1946, p.iii), certain 'operational links' may develop between these psychosomatic roles, integrating them into a unit, a sort of physiological self, or 'partial self'.[1]

Through a gradual differentiation between the child (the I) and his environment (the other - persons and objects), and between reality and fantasy, another two role categories emerge: the psychodramatic and the social roles. According to Moreno, these are connected to specific functions of the self: the psychodramatic roles allow the infant to experience the 'psyche'; while the social roles allow him to experience 'society' (psychosomatic roles helped the infant to experience the 'body'). With the appearance of these two role conglomerates, 'new forms of role playing are emerging, which correlate the infant to persons, things and goals in an actual setting outside of himself [social roles], and to persons, objects and goals which he *imagines* are outside of him [psychodramatic roles]' (Moreno 1946, p.73).

By the time he reaches the age of three, through the integration of the precursory, psychosomatic, social and psychodramatic roles, the child develops an ego, which will allow him to relate to others. Moreno (1923, p.8) writes:

> It is difficult to agree as to the structure of the self. I have described it as a cluster of roles (private plus collective roles). It reaches out beyond the skin of the individual organism; one of the 'beyonds' is the interpersonal realm. How far does it stretch and where does it end, is the question.

Based on his role theory, Moreno has also formulated a psychopathological view. According to him, psychosis is mainly a social condition, the psychotic as an individual being disconnected from his environment (social atom).

> We will frequently find some sort of disequilibrium within the different role groupings, that is, within the area of the psychosomatic or social roles, and even between these areas. This disequilibrium can lead to a delay in the emergence of the real self or the self as it is experienced; it can also intensify the disturbances of the self. (Moreno 1946, p.74)

As we will see in the following, some of the central ideas of the 'nucleus of the I' theory have had their origins in the above-presented Morenian concepts; some others however, were created and introduced by Bermudez. However, while in Moreno's view the development of the self (beyond the roles) is also strongly related to the concepts of spontaneity[2] and tele, Bermudez did not include these concepts in his own theory.

Bermudez's 'nucleus of the I' theory

Bermudez developed his 'nucleus of the I' theory by combining psychodramatic, psychoanalytic and physiological concepts. The two basic pillars of this theory are Moreno's concept of the psychosomatic roles, and Pichon-Riviere's theory of area integration. The 'nucleus of the I' is a theory of development and psychopathology that intended to extend and expand the psychodrama theory and technique, and through the understanding of the structure of the I, to create a bridge between the intra-psychic and the inter-relational. In the following I will present four of the most important aspects of Bermudez's theory.

The role structure

In the 'nucleus of the I' theory, the role structure (also referred to as the structure of the personality) is one the most crucial reference points. Bermudez represented the role structure in the graphic shape of a star (see Figure 5.1), with the nucleus of the I (14) at its centre. This nucleus is surrounded by the I (2) from which rays of different lengths beam out; it is as if the I would project out from this nucleus in relation to the world and itself. Thus the I envelops the nucleus of the I (or natural I), while on its outer periphery it is in contact with the social I.

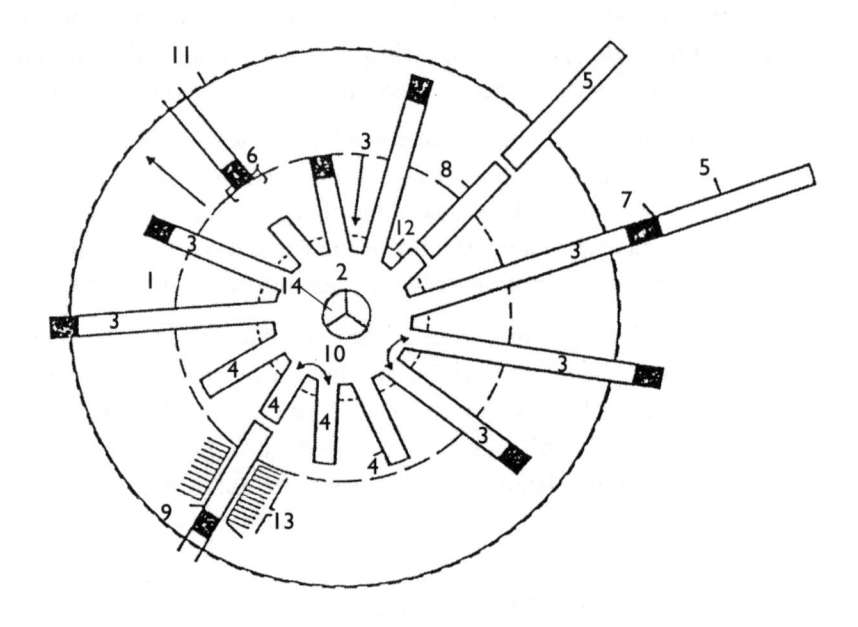

Figure 5.1 The role structure. 1 – The boundary of the self; 2 – The I; 3 – Roles; 4 – Underdeveloped role; 5 – Complementary role; 6 – Relationship between a complementary role and the boundary of the self; 7 – Link; 8 – Intermediary object; 9 – Pseudo-role; 10 – Relationship between roles; 11 – Expansion of the boundary of the self in an alarm state; 12 – Contraction of the boundary of the self in special warm-up situations; 13 – Context that maintains a pseudo-role; 14 – The nucleus of the I (Source: Rojas-Bermudez 1997, reproduced with permission)

The rays emerging from the I represent the social roles (3, 4) performed by an individual during his life. It is through these roles that the I relates to the complementary roles of the other (5) (for example, father–son or therapist–client), thus creating links (7) (for example, filial or therapeutic links). Bermudez differentiates between well developed roles (3) that will stretch beyond the boundary of the self (1), and underdeveloped roles (4), situated inside the area delineated by the boundary of the self. The more developed a role is, the more easily it will link with its complementary role. In the case of underdeveloped roles however, establishing links with the complementary roles is more difficult; these roles manifest or show themselves only when the boundary of the self is in a contracted state (12).

In Bermudez's role diagram this boundary of the self is represented by a dotted circle (1); he perceived it as a flexible and elastic membrane that envelops the I, representing the boundary between the I and the other. As the psychological boundary of the personality, it has a protective function, and in this respect is closely related to defence mechanisms. On a physical level, it corresponds to the peri-corporal (or personal) space, which every individual needs in order to feel at ease in the proximity of others. Experimentally, it can be verified by slowly approaching a person, checking where the point is when he/she starts to feel uncomfortable with the proximity of the other. For every individual there is a minimum distance to which he/she feels comfortable to be approached. This distance will vary in accordance with the psychological moment (circumstances) of the encounter, and with the stimuli involved. When the other (person) enters or invades the personal or peri-corporal space of the individual, a sense of discomfort is experienced. In other words, this happens when the role of an other (5) makes contact with the boundary of the self (6) and the individual does not have an appropriate complementary role (3) to establish a link. In this situation the individual may physically withdraw or push the other away. Psychologically, in a dramatization for example, the individual will get out of role or may do an irrational acting out.

The boundary of the self is not rigid, but it changes depending on the conditions (psychological moment) the individual is in. In a state of alarm or alertness (produced by either external or internal stimuli), this boundary expands (11), increasing its surface; under extreme circumstances this expansion may be to such a great extent, that the boundary of the self will cover up the roles (for example, in panic). In such a situation the individual will not only link through some of his roles, but in a more extended form through his whole being. In a more relaxed state on the other hand, the boundary of the self contracts, thus allowing roles to emerge and link. At times, the boundary can contract so much (in a sexual encounter for example [12]) that it gets in contact with the I (situated at the nucleus of the role structure).

Linking and links (7) are very important in the role development process, and are necessary in order to allow underdeveloped roles to emerge and to link with their complementary roles. The contraction of the boundary of the self (in a psychodrama session achieved through the warm-up) gives an opportunity for underdeveloped roles to become more visible, and so to be worked with psychodramatically.

In case of chronic psychotic clients the boundary of the self is permanently expanded. Bermudez worked extensively with psychotic clients, and through the use of puppets he developed the concept of the 'intermediary object' which will be presented later on.

The nucleus of the I

We saw that the 'nucleus of the I' is at the centre of the role structure described by Bermudez. He defines it as being 'a theoretical, genetic and structural framework, integrating the biological, psychological and social factors that play an important role in the individualization of the human being'[3] (Rojas-Bermudez 1997, p. 346).

Based on this initial definition, Bermudez assumes that at birth the child has a unique physiological sense of existence (related to his/her physiological functions), this being the first psychological manifestation of the organism.

These vital physiological functions are related to psychosomatic roles. Psychosomatic roles are based in the complementarity of the *internally programmed genetic structures* and the *externally programmed genetic structures* which are involved in the individual's matrix of identity, and are characteristic of our species. The infant is born with a set of necessities or needs that under normal circumstances are satisfied by the environment. These needs of the infant constitute what Bermudez called the *internally programmed genetic structures* (for example, the need for thermal, kinetic, tactile or sound stimuli). The responses provided by the environment that satisfy the child's needs are called the *externally programmed genetic structures* (for example, milk, warm clothes, caresses, soothing, nourishment, etc.).

Figure 5.2 is a schematic representation of this complementarity between the internally (1) and externally (2) programmed genetic structures. This complementarity results in the forming of a *memory trace* (3). Beyond the interaction of the complementary structures, within this memory trace the corresponding emotional discharge of the interaction is also registered. In other words, the way in which the developing child experiences his/her physiological needs and their resolutions (not just on an organic, but also on a relational level) will create psychological patterns of functioning. From the interaction between the biological structures (physiological needs) and the environmental structures (the resolution of these needs), memory traces result which will generate psychological manifestations (psychosomatic roles). The three vital physiological functions in which the psychosomatic roles originate, are ingestion, defecation and urination. The psychosomatic roles are named accordingly: the role of the ingestor, the role of the defecator and the role of the urinator.

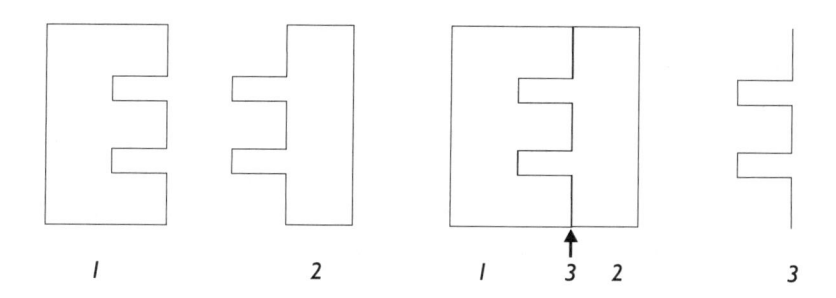

Figure 5.2 The complementarity of the internally and externally programmed genetic structures. 1 – Internally programmed genetic structure; 2 – Externally programmed genetic structure; 3 – Memory trace (Source: Rojas-Bermudez 1997, reproduced with permission)

The nucleus of the I develops from the *physiological self*, a term designated by Bermudez to describe this physiological sense of existence, characteristic of the new-born child; it can be seen as the total confusion (undifferentiation) between *mind*, *body* and *environment*. Bermudez represents the physiological self by a circle (Figure 5.3), however he adds that considering that a

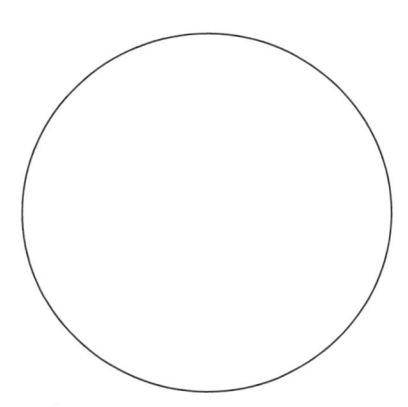

Figure 5.3 The physiological self (Source: Rojas-Bermudez 1997, reproduced with permission)

new-born baby has no limits, a graphic representation without limits would be more appropriate. The development (structuring) of the psychosomatic roles is fundamental to the progressive delimitation of the three areas (mind, body and environment). The delimitation and separation of these areas is exactly what will help the child solve the confusion of the chaotic and undifferentiated world (into which he was born), allowing him/her to develop a more complex social structure.

So, what Bermudez calls the 'nucleus of the I' is a structure resulting from the integration (or structuring) of the three psychosomatic roles (ingestor, defecator and urinator) with the three areas of the physiological self (mind, body and environment).[4] Graphically the 'nucleus of the I' is represented by a circle (the physiological self) divided into three equal slices by three radii (Figure 5.4). Each slice corresponds to an area and each radius corresponds to a psychosomatic role. The role of the *ingestor* (1) delimits the areas of the body (5) and the environment (4); the role of the *defecator* (2) delimits the areas of the mind (6) and environment (4); while the role of the *urinator* (3) delimits the areas of the mind (6) and body (5). From an evolutional perspective, the ingestor role develops in the first few months of the extra-uterine life; the defecator role develops between the third and eighth months of life; while the role of the urinator develops between the eighth and the twenty-fourth months of the child's life.

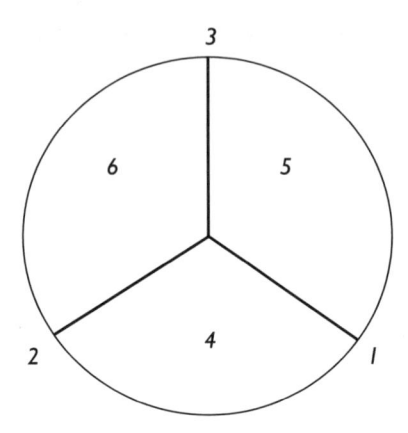

Figure 5.4 The nucleus of the I. Key: 1 – Ingestor role; 2 – Defecator role; 3 – Urinator role; 4 – Environment area; 5 – Body area; 6 – Mind area (Source: Rojas-Bermudez 1997, reproduced with permission)

The different developmental phases of the psychosomatic roles, determine different *psychosomatic models* (Figure 5.5). A psychosomatic model is more complex than simply the role(s) that it includes. Beyond including the corresponding role(s), it also includes all the external experiences that had occurred during the development of the role. For example, a surgical intervention during the first three months of life becomes an 'inheritance' of the ingestor role and so it becomes part of the ingestor model; if this intervention happens at one year of age, this experience will be incorporated into the urinator role and accordingly the urinator model.

The ingestor model:
1 – Ingestor role
2 – Physiological self

The defecator model:
1 – Ingestor role
2 – Defecator role
3 – Environment area
4 – Physiological self (mind and body still undifferentiated)

The urinator model:
1 – Ingestor role
2 – Defecator role
3 – Urinator role
4 – Environment area
5 – Body area
6 – Mind area

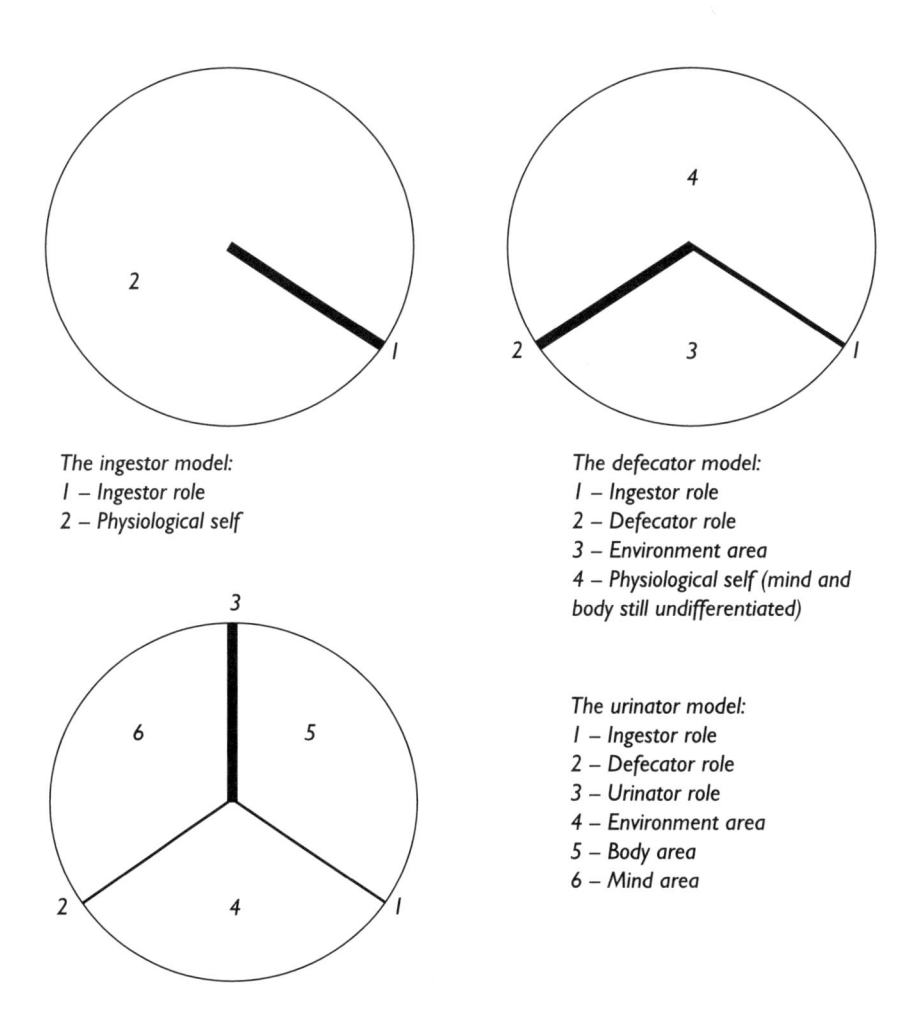

Figure 5.5 The psychosomatic models as described by Rojas-Bermudez (1997)

During the development period of the 'nucleus of the I', children receive different stimuli and stimulations, producing structures that later on will manifest themselves in the performance of roles. Since these stimuli may differ from child to child, every individual will develop roles that are specific for him/herself and that differ from roles developed by others; these roles are performed in a way characteristic to that particular individual.

Physio-psychopathology

In relation to mental illness, Bermudez (Rojas-Bermudez 1984, 1997) introduced the term *physio-psychopathology*. He differentiates between alterations of the psyche that originate in the role structure (psychopathology), and those that originate in the nucleus of the I (physio-psychopathology).

When describing the structure of the psychosomatic roles, Bermudez introduced the concept of *internally programmed genetic structures* (needs), which for their ideal development would need an adequate environment (or *externally programmed genetic structures*). As it was mentioned above, if a complementarity occurs between these internally and externally programmed genetic structures (that is the child's needs are met by the environment), this will result in the establishment of memory traces (see Figure 5.2). However, the lack of a definite or long-lasting complementarity will result in the fact that the memory trace will be incomplete or altered, presenting a gap (Figure 5.6) that Bermudez denominated *porosity* or *diathesis*. This gap in the memory trace (psychosomatic role) leads to the confusion of the areas delimited by the role (Figure 5.7).

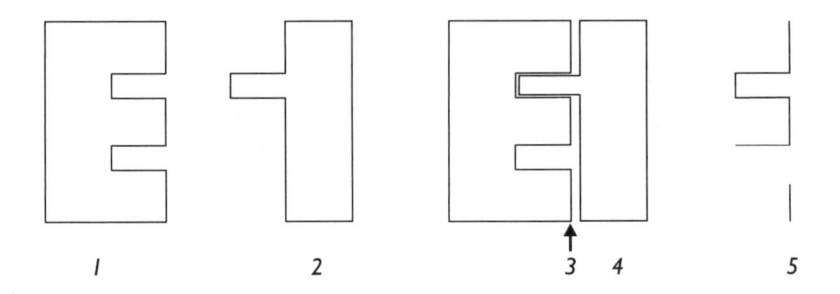

Figure 5.6 Porosity in the memory trace (psychosomatic role). 1 – Internally programmed genetic structure; 2 – Externally programmed genetic structure; 3 – Memory trace; 4 – Unsatisfactory externally programmed genetic structure; 5 – Porosity (or diathesis) in the memory trace (Source: Rojas-Bermudez 1997, reproduced with permission)

In Bermudez's view this confusion is at the basis of mental illness, or in other words, the confusion between the affected areas is considered as a primary symptom. When a porosity occurs in a psychosomatic role, the confusion resulting from this will generate *reparatory mechanisms* (secondary symptoms) in order to maintain the equilibrium of the I. The reparatory mechanism will emerge as a result of the tension accumulated within the unsatisfied (deprived) internally programmed genetic structure. For example: the lack of physical contact during the development of the ingestor role, will lead to an accumulation of tension on a cutaneos level (skin), which will motivate the creation of a corresponding reparatory mechanism (Figure 5.7, A).

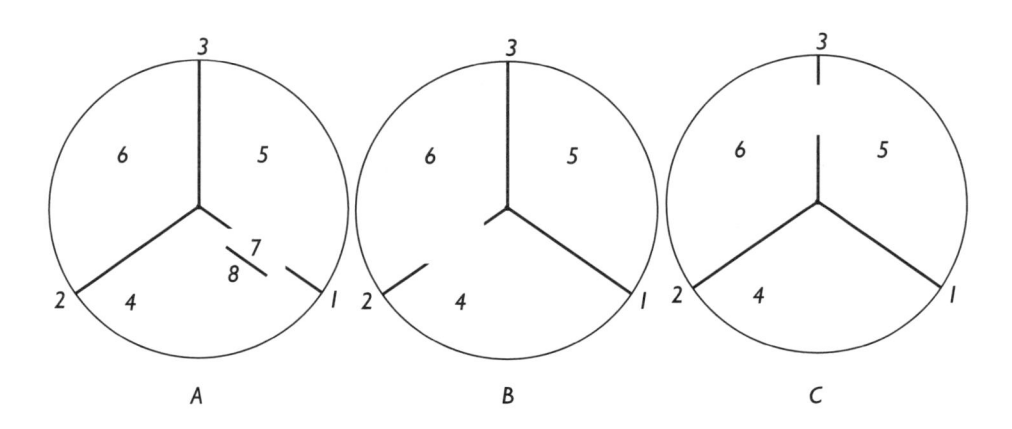

Figure 5.7 Porosities of the psychosomatic roles. A – Porosity of the ingestor role; B – Porosity of the defecator role; C – Porosity of the urinator role. 1 – Ingestor role; 2 – Defecator role; 3 – Urinator role; 4 – The environment area; 5 – The body area; 6 – The mind area; 7 – Porosity (or diathesis); 8 – Reparatory mechanism (Source: Rojas-Bermudez 1997, reproduced with permission)

Bermudez (Rojas-Bermudez 1984) described reparatory mechanisms as dynamic activities and classified them in the following way:

- Porosity of the ingestor role:
    ◦ phobic hysteria
    ◦ hysteric conversion.

- Porosity of the defecator role:
  - psychopathic personality
  - depression.
- Porosity of the urinator role:
  - obsessive ideas or thoughts
  - compulsive actions.

If the porosity appears during the development of the ingestor role, the confusion will appear between the areas of the body and environment, resulting in hysterical symptoms. Reparatory mechanisms originating on the environmental side will lead to phobic hysteria, while the reparatory mechanisms originating in the body area will lead to hysteric conversion.

If the porosity appears during the formation of the defecator role, this will lead to the confusion of the mind and the environment areas. The reparatory mechanisms on the side of the environmental area will lead to psychopathic personality, while the reparatory mechanisms in the mind area will lead to depression.

If the porosity appears during the formation of the urinator role, the confusion will be between the areas of the body and mind. The reparatory mechanisms on the side of the body area lead to compulsive rituals and actions, while reparatory mechanisms on the side of the mind area will lead to obsessive ideation and thoughts.

In all the above cases the porosity affects only one of the three psychosomatic roles, resulting in the confusion of two corresponding areas. Thus the third, intact area becomes hyper-functional. In Bermudez's view this hyperfunction of one of the three areas, corresponds to neurosis.

Psychosis, on the other hand, is the result of the porosity within two psycho-somatic roles, that is, the confusion of all three areas, leaving the individual with only one intact psycho-somatic role that will become hyper-functional. According to Bermudez, while the porosities are seen as the primary symptoms, the reparatory mechanisms (produced to fill in the porosities) are considered as secondary symptoms of psychosis. The confusion between the areas, jointly with the reparatory mechanisms, will lead to psychotic behaviour or states.

The porosities of the psychosomatic roles often are repaired; as a result the individual will adapt to a complementary social atom, and will continue his development through this adaptive structure. However, if reparatory mechanisms are insufficient and so fail to repair the porosities, the confusion between the areas will persist, effecting the structuring (development) of roles, the individual's psychological contact with his environment, as well as his relationship with himself.

The boundary of the self is intimately connected to the emotions and the defence mechanisms of the I. In stressful situations (provoking an alarm state in the individual) the boundary of the self will expand and will cover up all the well developed roles. These alarm states can be acute or chronic. The acute states of alarm correspond to states of panic, while the chronic ones to psychotic states. In case of psychosis, the chronic expansion of the boundary will lead to the individual's alienation from his environment and his disconnection from his social atom. The individual will live enclosed in his own world; he will perceive any approach from outside as threatening, because he does not have roles available to respond (his roles cannot stretch beyond the expanded boundary of the self). Possible responses to this are mutism, negativism, or delirium, among others.

The symptoms will depend on the intact (hyper-functional) role. Bermudez describes the following three possibilities:

1. If the ingestor role is intact, this will lead to a hyper-function of the ingestor model, resulting in the dominance of incorporative mechanisms (the individual's attempt to 'ingest' or 'swallow' the whole environment) as well as reparatory mechanisms characteristic of the porosities of the urinator and defecator roles (see above). This corresponds to the clinical picture of melancholy as described in classic psychiatry.

2. If the defecator role is intact, there will be a hyper-function of this model. This will lead to confusion between thinking, feeling and environment, resulting in the dominance of 'productive' mechanisms, corresponding to the delirant clinical pictures of classic psychiatry. It will also be accompanied by reparatory mechanisms characteristic of the porosities of the urinator and ingestor roles.

3. If the urinator role is intact, and so hyper-functional, the internal confusion of the individual will be transposed to the external world in the form of action, resulting in behaviour that corresponds to the manic clinical pictures described in classic psychiatry. Reparatory mechanisms characteristic of the porosities of the ingestor and defecator role will be also present.

In all three of the above situations there is confusion in the individual's feelings, thoughts and actions.

Looking at psychosis from a phenomenological perspective, Bermudez has also introduced a distinction between two fundamental psychotic alterations: those that manifest themselves in the individual's relation to space, and those that manifest themselves in the individual's relation to time. In the case of so-called *spatial psychosis* the individual perceives his surroundings in an unstructured and disintegrated way. Psychosis will de-structure (fragment) the images from the individual's environment to such an extent that he will be unable to gain a holistic view of these, and, as a result these images will become persecuting (in Bermudez's terminology *monstrous images*). In the case of the *temporal psychosis*, it is the individual's ability to form a sequence of situations (scenes) that is perturbed, affecting his perception of past, present and future. As a consequence, in both cases an alarm state develops, the boundary of the self expands, the individual disconnects and becomes alienated from his social network. Self-absorption and delirium can be seen as the individual's attempts to protect the self from a greater de-structuring and total disintegration.

While Moreno described psychosis mainly as a social condition, and the psychotic client as an individual disconnected from his environment, in his understanding of the self and psychosis, Bermudez has also introduced physiological and psychological elements (beyond the social aspect). He describes psychosis on the following three levels:

1. On a social level – as an absence of roles, with the consequence of the individual's disconnection from the environment.

2. On a physiological level – in Bermudez's view, the integrity of the psychosomatic roles is a result of the individual's physiological experiences; the structure (development) of the psychosomatic roles is conditioned by the complementarity of the externally and internally programmed genetic structures. In the absence of this complementarity confusion appears between the areas, leading to psychotic symptoms.

3. On a psychological level – he defines the psychotic as an individual with the boundary of his self chronically expanded, covering up all his roles (this explains the absence of roles); this expansion is due to the confusion of the three areas.

These physiological and psychological re-definitions of the psychosis result from Bermudez's conception regarding the psychological evolutional development of the individual, in which he systematizes the concept of the I through the psychosomatic roles.

The intermediary object

Bermudez developed the term *intermediary object* through his work with chronic psychotic clients, while using puppets and marionettes in order to attract their attention during psychodrama sessions.[5] He observed the enormous power of attraction of the puppets and also their positive influence during warm-up. Warm-up with his psychotic patients usually took up to 30 to 40 minutes, but happened in 5 to 10 minutes when using puppets. Beyond simply just capturing the patients' attention, Bermudez also discovered that puppets were very valuable tools of communication.

> During a group session one of the patients seemed to be hallucinating. I approached this patient to question him, but all my efforts were useless, since I didn't manage to pull a single word out of him. So, I turned all my attention to the rest of the group. Later on, I asked one of my trained auxiliaries (who was working with puppets) to approach this patient and try to talk to him and ask the same questions for which I did not manage to get answers. A puppet appeared on the scene, and after a brief monologue, directed itself to the patient calling him by his name. The patient observed carefully and responded. Soon after, a dialogue developed between the puppet and the patient, and he answered all the questions without resistance, showing signs of sympathy towards the puppet. (Rojas-Bermudez 1977, p.93)

> A patient with intense auditory hallucinations regularly interrupted the scenes, but without any apparent participation in what was going on in the group. We tried many different ways to communicate with him, however, only obtained some of his conventional phrases. He usually submerged in his hallucinations and withdrew from the session. One day a puppet called him by the name and continued talking to him; the patient became very surprised, smiled and started a conversation with the puppet. Following this first contact with the puppet, a radical change took place in the patient's attitude. He didn't just become attentive towards the dramatizations, but started to regularly participate in them, initially only through the mediation of the puppets and later on with the trained auxiliaries. (Rojas-Bermudez 1977, p.94)

According to Bermudez, what is important in the above examples is the fact that with the puppets they obtained a response that couldn't be obtained through an attempt at direct, person-to-person contact with the client. However, the clients responded when the emitter of the message was not human. Through a deeper investigation Bermudez observed a similar phenomenon in situations when the client was in intense alarm, or alterations of the corporal scheme.

The common denominator in all these situations was the fear or threat of being invaded by the emitter (with human characteristics). The puppets on the other hand (an emitter which doesn't have the same characteristics), were perceived by the patients as harmless and innocuous objects, and therefore could be used therapeutically. Based on its quality of being an object and its function of mediation, Bermudez denominated it *intermediary object*. (In his diagram of the role structure [Figure 5.1] the intermediary object is numbered 8.)

Regarding the relationship between the intermediary object and the boundary of the self in the above-presented examples, Bermudez states that the alertness kept the patients' boundary of self expanded to such an extent, that this did not allow the occurrence of links (role/counter-role relationships). Through the use of the puppets as intermediary objects, a certain degree of warm-up was achieved that allowed the emergence of roles and the establishment of links. Bermudez concludes that in case of very underdeveloped roles, puppets (as unthreatening objects) allow a communication through their ability to penetrate the boundary of the self without causing an alarm reaction; a characteristic that allows a therapeutic use of puppets (role–intermediary object–role relation).[6]

The therapeutic use of the intermediary object however, is not reduced only to serious mental illness but, according to Bermudez, can be applied in all those cases when we work with underdeveloped roles and/or alarm states (that keep the boundary of the self expanded). There are further situations when the use of intermediary objects is also recommended by Bermudez, even when the actual role is well developed. These are situations when certain aspects of the dramatized role may unchain an unexpected alarm reaction, which the protagonist cannot control. Generally speaking these are scenes that involve aggressive or erotic roles.

According to Bermudez, when working with functional roles, intermediary objects can also be used as stimulation to make evident or to demonstrate certain unconscious aspects or conflicting behaviours that are avoided.

> A psychodrama training group reached a very competitive phase, but without any manifestations of rivalry in relation to the director. During

one of the dramatizations the director placed a handkerchief on the floor without any explanation. The dramatization continued, but slowly became focused on the handkerchief. At a certain point the five characters of the drama were sat in a circle around the handkerchief, introducing this new element into the dramatization. One of them started to warm his hands as it would have been a fireplace; a second one kicked it away; the third picked it up, examined it and then pretended to blow his nose; the fourth one crumpled it up like an old piece of paper, while the last smoothened it out, pretending it was a tablecloth. The others responded to this by improvising a picnic. All of them were praising the food, until someone noticed that ants were crawling over it, blaming another for not taking care of the food. Two others also started to complain about the food not being seasoned. A discussion broke out regarding the responsibilities of each member. The fifth, who did not say anything, started to gather the tablecloth, keeping it for himself. The others, trying to take the tablecloth from him, eventually ripped it, an event that stopped the action, since none of them knew what to do. (Rojas-Bermudez 1977, p.100)

Bermudez points out how the stimulus (the object of the director) evoked different responses in the protagonists; how spontaneous changes occurred in the dramatization as a result of the interactions with this intermediary object; and the manifest link of the dramatization with the therapist. He also draws the attention to the warm-up effect of the intermediary object within this case: the participants got so deeply involved in the situation, that they ended up acting without their observer I.

Bermudez summarizes the following eight important characteristics of the intermediary object as a therapeutic tool:

1. It has a real and concrete existence.
2. It is harmless (it does not unchain alarm responses per se).
3. It is malleable (it can be used at ease in any complementary role play).
4. It is characterized by transmissivity: it allows communication by substituting the link and maintaining the distance between the complementary roles.
5. Adaptability: it is adapted to the needs of the individual.
6. Assimilability: it allows such an intimate relationship, that the individual can identify it with himself.

7. Instrumentality: it can be used as an extension of the individual.
8. Identificability: it can be easily recognized.

Final considerations

Using the Morenian role theory as his starting point, Bermudez developed an evolutional theory of the personality development, strongly emphasizing the interaction between the organism and the environment. Based on the somatic functions of alimentation, defecation and urination, he stressed the importance of role complementarity, and approaching man (and the psychotic client) in his social, psychological and physiological totality, he introduced a technique with a wide range of application.

During the 1970s and early 1980s the 'nucleus of the I' became one of the main theoretical reference points in the Brazilian psychodrama. While many professionals and psychodrama schools adhered to the 'Bermudian tradition', numerous others became more and more critical of this theory, gradually breaking away from it.

Today Bermudez lives and continues his work in Spain, and in a more recent publication (Rojas-Bermudez 1997) he has updated his theory with the latest results of neurophysiologic and brain research. When presenting this theory, my intention wasn't to discuss its validity or invalidity; what I was hoping to achieve within this chapter was an objective presentation of these ideas (if such thing is possible), placing Bermudez's theory in its historical context and recognizing its value and influence for the development of the Brazilian psychodrama movement. In my view, the greatest credit of Bermudez is his courage to break away from a dominant conserve (the Morenian theory) and – following also the Morenian principles of spontaneity and creativity – to attempt a further development of the psychodramatic project.

Notes

1 'Similarly, in the course of development, the psychodramatic roles begin to cluster and produce a sort of psychodramatic self, and finally, the social roles begin to cluster and form a sort of social self. The physiological, psychodramatic and social selves are only "part" selves; the really integrated, entire self, of later years is still far from being born' (Moreno 1946, p.iii).
2 'My thesis is, the locus of self is spontaneity' (Moreno 1923, p.8).

3   According to Moreno (1923, p.8): 'The self is the melting pot of experiences coming from many directions. One of the dimensions of the self is the social, another dimension is the sexual, another is the biological,...but it is more than any one of them.'

4   This idea is similar to what Moreno wrote in 'Psychodrama' (1946, p.iii): 'Body, psyche and society are the intermediary parts of the entire self.'

5   Influenced by a technique called 'symbolic realization' introduced by Marguerite Seschèhaye (1947), Pierre Bour (in France) has also used objects with symbolic values in his work with chronic schizophrenic clients (Altenfelder 2001).

6   As mentioned above, in spatial psychosis, clients experience a disintegration of the images they perceive. Bermudez has also used intermediary objects in his attempt to help psychotic clients re-structure these fragmented images. While in cases of temporal psychosis he applied so-called 'intermediary situations' in order to help clients recover their sense of temporality and integrate present, past and future in a coherent continuum. Intermediary situations are scenes that mediate between the internal images of the patient and the reality as experienced in the psychodrama. In this respect, both the intermediary objects and the intermediary situations work with the capacity of understanding the environment as a structural whole (Gestalt).

6

The clusters theory[1]

Dalmiro M. Bustos

Introduction

It was in 1990 that I formulated the first concepts of the 'clusters theory' (Bustos 1990, 1994), and upon revisiting it I realized that an update was necessary. Over the last few years, I have worked a great deal on this theory, which allowed me to further expand and modify many concepts. Therefore, I decided to rewrite this text and share my current vision on this subject.

In couples therapy, group therapy, as well as individual therapy, clear references are needed in order to help us understand the everyday dynamics of the human being. The wonderful classical descriptions refer to neurotic, psychotic and character-pathologic cases. However, in our psychotherapy work we often deal with the dynamics of relationship problems that do not fit into these traditional descriptions. In the following I will try to convey to the reader certain parameters that will allow us to understand the human being through a perspective that is not focused on pathology; I will focus instead on all those dynamics that are found in the grey areas, and cannot be characterized within the classical frameworks, but reflect the various angles of human suffering. In other words, I will focus on that unstable equilibrium called normality. My starting point is Moreno's interpersonal theory.

The initial concepts of Moreno and further developments based on his teachings

Moreno (1946) defines the roles as being the tangible and real aspects the Ego takes. However, being concise and systematic are certainly not among Moreno's many and valuable virtues. As a result, there are numerous contradictions within his extensive work that may lead to confusion. I shall only mention the most significant one, in which the role is defined as a psycho-social behavioural unit. Every role is a fusion of private and collective elements, which Moreno defines as 'collective denominators and individual differentials' (Moreno 1934). The role concept represents the central axis of his theory, the point of departure for all his considerations. Moreno developed his theory of interpersonal relations based on this concept. 'Roles are not isolated; they tend to form clusters. There is a transfer of s [spontaneity] from unenacted roles to the presently enacted ones. This influence is called *cluster effect*' (Moreno 1946, p.175).

This affirmation has evoked a question in me: is it possible to understand the human soul and its sufferings based on this special role-grouping – what Moreno called cluster? If the experiences of the human being are transmitted to all the roles, these experiences impregnating the roles, then, observing the roles in interaction (the inter-psychic in Moreno's words) should also allow us to understand the internal dynamics (the intra-psychic in Moreno's words). In order to follow this path, I will first briefly make some references to the developmental process, as described by Moreno.

The matrix of identity

> Co-being, co-action and co-experience, which, in the primary phase exemplify the infant's relationship to the persons and things around him, are characteristics of the *matrix of identity*. This matrix of identity lays the foundation for the first emotional learning process of the infant. (Moreno 1946, p.61)

Following this direct reference to Moreno, I will present my own elaborations based on his teachings. I believe that Moreno's essential spirit will reflect through my thoughts; however, it is not my intention to stay faithful to him – I just want to do what he always taught me: to be creative.

The above-mentioned Morenian concepts are essential in order to understand the intra-psychic development. Everything that surrounds the infant – especially his mother, being the closest person with whom he shares his world – is part of the infant. What happens around him is experienced as if it happened inside him. The burden of tensions of the family environment surrounding the infant will become a constituent part of him, impregnating the infant. The infant doesn't have the ability to discriminate between the Ego (I) and non-Ego (non-I). This discrimination is an ego function that will only develop later.

This primary phase will strongly define the infant's subsequent development: 'the world is, and I am: hard, tense, receptive, accessible, aggressive, etc.' It generates an anticipation of how he will think about the world and vice-versa. Since these first experiences are not filtered through a psychic apparatus – because this does not exist yet – they have a very powerful and irrefutable impact on the infant.

The maternal function of feeding the baby generates a first behaviour, essential for the infant's survival. This is the infant's first role, born out of the mother–child relationship and the need to be supplied with the necessary nourishment. According to the developmental sequence proposed by Moreno, this is the first role that will start to outline the Ego. Moreno calls these first roles 'psychosomatic', since they depend on the essential functions for survival and they are not performed based on desire but out of a biological need. In my view, the so-called psychosomatic roles are biologically determined functions such as urination, breathing, alimentation and defecation. The infant accomplishes these functions with the help of the mother or the adult who takes on this task. Therefore, they are functions derived from the mother–child roles, or *protoroles*. The only function among those mentioned above that does not require the mother's auxiliary presence, is breathing.

Subsequent learning will open the doors for autonomous functions such as locomotion, babbling and talking.

The structure of the Ego will develop through the internalization of the rules that are in force within the environment in which the infant develops. This takes place through the intermediation of the parents. The infant will learn the rules of the game, and will start to anticipate them. Not too long ago – due to the belief that this was a healthy practise – babies used to be wrapped up tightly, in order to keep their spine straight. Later on, this myth was replaced by another practise of leaving the baby as loose as possible, without being bound. Habits vary according to the actual knowledge, and myths are replaced by other myths, depending on the values that are in force within a certain era. Similarly, opinions regarding how to feed the baby also often change; the idea of feeding the baby strictly every three or four hours and let him cry in order to learn a 'healthy' rhythm, gave way to another feeding rhythm determined by the infant's hunger. Learning the rules that anticipate the behaviour will structure the psychic instance called the Ego. This structuring process happens through the role of the infant (whose central dynamic is that of being fed) and the complementary role of the mother (or her substitute). However, whoever fulfils this function is perceived by the infant as the same person, because his perception is not mature enough biologically in order to distinguish the difference between persons performing this function.

As the infant grows, he will have other needs; someone to help him stand, to reach objects. From being an involuntary act, fulfilling his needs becomes an act of will. This phase of the development is related to the paternal function. We also know that conventionally this is more strongly determined by culture than biology: according to the traditional model, the paternal function is performed by the father; however, it can also be performed by the mother or any other adult within the child's environment. From the infant's perspective, his role continues to be that of the child. Nevertheless, it is called the paternal function, even if it can be performed by a woman. Some years ago, this explanation would not have been relevant. However, the accepted models of couples have significantly changed since: today, two men or two women in a homosexual relationship can adopt babies and perform the functions that before had been strictly reserved to a biological condition. The only function that cannot be modified is pregnancy; a function related only to women, for the time being.

So, the Ego will accumulate the rules of the game of the society in which it develops. Spontaneity – being in the centre of the human being's vital functions – will be 'filtered' through these rules, which will guide it, constituting the ego function of *adequacy*, considered by Moreno as a quality of spontaneity. Without this filter that contains the rules considered desirable by a society, spontaneity would be only spontaneism.

Subsequently, the third central role appears: the role of the sibling, a role that once again we should refer to as a function. Even those who do not have any brothers or sisters will find in their social atom cousins or friends, equals that require new behaviour. The appearance of this third central role will expand the child's universe with new family roles. He has already learnt to differentiate between objects and persons, fantasies and reality, what happens inside or outside of him. Between me and not-me. He is already prepared to start on the risky path towards adult life.

As a result, the Ego will develop another of its central functions: that of selecting roles. Each interaction is carried out through the appropriate role: that of the son, brother, grandson, nephew, friend, student, etc. Each role will have its special characteristics as well as common denominators. And it is the Ego that will select and adapt the roles and the corresponding behaviour. The exchange of experiences happens through the cluster effect.

Clusters

The above introduction was aimed to sequentially order the Morenian ideas in order to help us understand the cluster concept. As the central nervous system matures, the capacity of the human memory – that is, the capacity to register and accumulate experiences – also develops. The experiences of the human being are structured by emotions and later on images. Goleman (1996) offers us an understanding of the actions, full of myths and entanglements between the psychological and the biological. He writes: 'In the everyday life there is no intelligence more important than the interpersonal intelligence.' Without directly referring to him, Goleman's thoughts regarding the 'inter-personal' coincide with that of Moreno's: 'A life without passion would be a boring desert, remote and separated from the richness of life. But, as Aristotle pointed out, what we want is an adequate emotion, to feel in harmony with the circumstances' (Goleman 1996).

Here, another Morenian concept – adequacy, as the fundamental condition of spontaneity – is again presented from the perspective of emotional intelligence, unfortunately though, without mentioning Moreno's pioneering contributions. However, if we put this omission aside, we can see that Goleman accomplishes one of Moreno's dreams: to find the biological bases of the concept of spontaneity:

> LeDoux's investigations elucidate how the tonsil can exercise control over what we do, even while the neo-cortex (the thinking brain), is trying to make a decision. As we will see, the functioning of the tonsil and its interaction with the neo-cortex are right at the core of the emotional intelligence.
>
> Certain emotional reactions and emotional memories may form without the slightest cognitive and conscious involvement. The tonsil can harbour response registers and repertoires, responses that we perform without knowing exactly why we perform them; this is due to the fact that the shortcut from the thalamus to the tonsil avoids the neo-cortex completely. It seems that this bypass makes it possible for the tonsil to become a *deposit of emotional impressions and memories* [the italics are mine], of which we were never totally conscious. (Goleman 1996)

These affirmations help us to better understand Reich's concepts regarding the bodily memory and Moreno's concept of spontaneity, demystifying them in order to integrate pathological and biological investigations.

Returning to the subject of clusters, when Moreno writes that roles exchange their experiences, he means that they are grouped according to certain dynamics. My question was: what is the criterion based on which roles form these role-groupings? From an evolutionary perspective we may think that during each phase the infant incorporates experiences that will strongly influence his future development. From this point of view we can divide this learning process into three groups: cluster one, with the complementary role of the mother (or the adult that substitutes her); cluster two, with the complementary role of the father (or his adult replacement), and cluster three, with the complementary role of the sibling (or his equivalents).

Cluster one: maternal cluster

As it was already mentioned, the infant is born in a state of complete defencelessness: if he does not get help, he dies. Unlike many other species that are born with a sufficient maturity to survive, the human infant is born unable to be autonomous; he is neither biologically nor psychologically able to survive without help. When mentioning the matrix of undifferentiated all-identity, I also said that the baby experiences everything that happens around him as if it was a part of him. The body registers the tensions and incorporates them as their own. The infant is especially sensitive to the distress of the people around him. The secure or insecure holding of the mother's arms will determine an anticipation of tenderness and calmness or of anxiety and tension in connection with the care the infant receives. The key word for this developmental phase is *dependency* and the complementary role is that of the *mother*.

For our later performance in the adult life, it is essential to learn to be dependent. The abilities to receive, to accept being taken care of, and to live together healthily during moments of vulnerability, are based on the experiences of this phase. Let us consider breastfeeding: if the mother does this in a positive way – her desire to have the baby extending into the pleasure of taking care of him and sharing with him the discovery of the world – then this energy will become a constituent part of the act of receiving. As a result, when the infant needs or lacks something, he will ask for it naturally and without feelings of guilt. His spontaneity will be filtered through this incorporated experience, allowing him access to an adequate response. The same is true for other dependent functions, for example personal hygiene. It is important that these are done efficiently, however what is fundamental is the way they are fulfilled.

The first primary emotion of the human being is inexorably connected to the sensations, *tenderness* being an important constituent of both. The term comes from tender, vulnerable. Often forgotten in psychology, it is not included in any classification, and so frequently left unnoticed, just as the concept of the soul. Without doubt however, the capacity to feel and accept tenderness is essential in order to develop *intimate* relationships. It also allows transgressing the distance in relationships that require greater emotional distance, as work relationships, for example. The mother's arms are the feeling they generate, the infant does not distinguish between them. Within the Latin cultures, tenderness has greater relational opportunities to manifest itself. Latin Americans tend to touch more, even if men (instead of hugging) prefer to pat one another on the back in order not to risk looking homosexual. Women however are much better in showing tenderness. Men also more readily give and receive tenderness from women, without the fear of homophobia. However, men also often sexualize the contact in order to be able to accept it: it is easier for a man to ask for sex than to ask for emotional contact. Both men and women however, need tenderness as a constituent part of intimate relationships. Without tenderness strength becomes toughness. The so-called sensitivity towards someone else's pain is loaded with feelings of tenderness. The ability to get close to someone without any feelings of threat, to respect the other and to show affability, have their matrix in the primary feeling of tenderness. If tenderness is replaced by the mere efficiency of the carers, this may leave indelible marks resulting in the fact that the person will tend to automate his emotional relationships. Generally speaking, tenderness does not require many words: it is pre-verbal and self-explanatory. By trying to put words to it, we may take away its depth. I would like to further add here, that if tenderness is not accompanied by the learning of boundaries, rules and autonomy, it may become a prison of extreme dependent relationships (attachment), or it could result in the opposite: its total denial (in order to avoid being at the mercy of the loved ones).

When emphasizing the importance of these first experiences, I do this mainly in relation to the initial matrix of *pleasure*. If within this phase the infant develops a pleasant and pleasurable anticipation in relation to alimentation and basic care, this anticipated pleasure will persist as a background for the subsequent experiences. It will become a quality that is present in the various aspects of life, whether it is making love, working or fulfilling an obligation. People with these characteristics are able to create a pleasant atmosphere and to positively impregnate their environment by their mere presence.

Self-esteem is strongly conditioned by this phase, just as *self-affirmation* depends on cluster two (paternal cluster). The glance of the mother, representing the glance of the infant's environment, will be the glance through which the infant will observe his own actions. Tenderness and receptivity anticipate a loving relationship with oneself. By loving I do not mean being complaisant and willing to justify everything, but being containing in order to accept mistakes. The fear of an excessively severe internal judgement will cause a flight from healthy self-criticism.

It is also important to remember that these situations are not merely determined by external influences, even if the infant cannot yet differentiate between what is internal and external. Freud's complementary sequences are valid and should not be forgotten when considering the formation of a person's characteristics. Genetic as well as exogenous factors can have both positive and negative influences, and they are absolutely interlinked and indivisible. We only separate them in order to gain a better understanding of them, or due to our inability to think in an integrated manner. Moreno (1946, p.52) describes them as factors linked to the g (genes), s (spontaneity), t (tele) and e (environment) functions.

While they do not yet form a psychic apparatus that mediates between the acquired primary experiences, these experiences have an extensive tensional register. Strictly speaking, the much discussed corporal memory can be understood as the most highly developed register of the infant: his body. Within an evolutionary sequence the tensional register develops first; this is followed by the development of the emotional register, and then the intellectual register. Memory traces require the development of the central nervous system; a system that is absent at birth. The act hunger referred to by Moreno, is an uninterrupted sequence of actions without any register or purpose. However, these actions are capable of perceiving tension.

Negative experiences of this cluster may greatly hinder later development. Abandonment and desertion – resulting in the lack of constituents for emotional survival – may lead to the human being's inability to move to the next developmental stage. Laing (1974) described this condition as the basic ontological insecurity. The lack of loving carers may undermine the infant's physical and psychological development; this may lead to psychosis or even death in more serious cases.

An overprotected infant is also learning about life and love. Attachment behaviour generally has its origins within primary contacts with an imprisoning quality. When I asked one of my patients who presented these characteristics what did love mean to him, he responded: 'it is something similar to glue; it is something that protects and supports you, but it also keeps you stuck to the beloved person.' Another patient smilingly said: 'a pretty and gentle flower; a carnation.' Carnation or clove pink is a parasite plant that dies together with its host.

The enormous power of primary learning lies within the fact that these experiences are recorded as *myths*, as *truths* that do not require confirmation. Their register takes place prior to the ability of reasoning. Socially, they represent the collective unconscious. They are installed into an unattainable place. In spite of the rudimentary ego, the *ego-syntony* indicates that all these stimuli are incorporated as belongings of a natural order. One of my patients told me that he was born after four involuntary abortions of his mother. Since his early childhood a fear of death has been haunting him. He always feels in danger and in spite of being an intelligent professional, he is not able to make the necessary efforts required by his professional practise. He feels that everything is beyond his strength and frequently talks about feeling 'broken'. He has an allergic rhinitis, which he sees as an irrefutable proof of his genetic weakness. The fear of his death actually belongs to his mother; however, in this particular moment of development this doesn't make any difference whatsoever.

In this primary state of defencelessness, the infant learns that hostility and abandonment, or on the contrary, overprotection are unchangeable; *the world is like this*, and *he is like this*. He learns that threat is continuously around and so he will have to implement certain means for survival. All human beings need to learn how to face the anxiety generated by the frustrations of life; this is generally achieved through behaviours that will allow emotional survival. The efficiency of this behaviour and the greater or smaller expense of its implementation will play an essential role in the positive or negative adaptation to the adult world. I would like to stress that *all human beings* resort to specific strategies to deal with anxiety; the greater the variety of resources, the greater the person's versatility. These are the so called *defence mechanisms*. Of course, nobody can surpass Anna Freud's meticulous work and Melanie Klein's contributions regarding the defence mechanisms. Considering however, that at the centre of their investigation is neurosis and psychosis, defence mechanisms remain impregnated with pathological concepts. And even if explicitly described by these authors, defence mechanisms are seen as belonging to the realm of neurosis and psychosis. However, this is not absolutely so. Anxiety is a feared characteristic of the human being, the counterpart of spontaneity; either of them only appears after overcoming the other. From the moment of birth, strategies must be implemented in order to assure emotional survival.

Dissociation is the first ordering factor within the chaos of the first universe. Repression ensures the adequacy of behaviour. According to Jorge Luis Borges, without dissociation and repression civilization would not exist. We structure our 'natural' characteristics as we learn to use new strategies. The duration and proportionality of the applied behaviours make the difference along the fine boundary that separates what is normal from what is pathological. The mechanism of adaptation can be seen as successful, when – in front of a negative stimulus that threatens our equilibrium – we are able to implement a resource, overcoming the threat. If this resource persists once the danger is gone, or the relation between the stimulus and the resource disappears, we are within the realm of pathology. Being paralysed or running away from a fire or an attack is not the same as becoming paralysed or running away from a harmless mouse. It may seem common sense, however I would like to point out that I consider this form of behaviour to be a strategy with negative effects for the patients. But, just as myths have a powerful effect of impregnation, common knowledge may also adapt certain concepts, transforming them into something that cannot be suppressed. When Freud's indivisible thoughts became public, they were distorted and trivialized. Thus, an orderly person is considered obsessive; someone who vividly expresses his feelings is considered hysterical; someone afraid of something is considered phobic, etc.

Within this developmental phase, a relationship with one's needs is built up: living together with them without anxiety ensures the possibility of not denying them, just as there is no human being who can establish a loving relationship without feeling that the beloved, besides being desired, is also needed. Mature dependency, a requisite for establishing a long-lasting relationship, often changes into primary and infantile need. Life doesn't evolve in a linear way. Nobody feels completely fulfilled throughout his life. And in these moments of failure, loss and fear of life, desire often becomes an imperative need. If someone has passed through the maternal cluster in a natural way, feeling well-cared for, he will be able to accept these moments. If this doesn't happen, it can bring a relationship to an end, even ending up hating the other person because of feeling that he/she is essential for the relationship.

The predominant *basic emotions* of this phase are *voracity* and *envy*. Melanie Klein (in Segal 1972) defines them as the most primary feelings of the human being. According to the above-described sequence, within the matrix of the undifferentiated all-identity, the infant's basic primary need is nourishment. If this need is unsatisfied, it will generate tension and anxiety, threatening the infant's survival. If deprivation is persistently accompanied by frustration, *voracity* will develop. Food will be consumed with hatred. Incorporating food becomes a dangerous act loaded with anxiety. The mere anticipation of the need for food may turn into an overwhelming threat. We could say that this voracity is more of a hate than hunger, destroying the person who needs to be fed.

Envy is the other basic emotion connected to this stage. Undoubtedly, it is one of the most destructive motives of human beings. From an evolutionary perspective envy develops after voracity. In the initial phase of the stage of undifferentiated all-identity the need to be fed and the source of food are the same thing. Therefore, this phase of identity is protected from envy, because one cannot envy what one owns. As a result of psycho-physical maturation, the infant will start to differentiate the world that surrounds him. The other and the I become divided and therefore the infant starts to become aware of the fact that the source of pleasure does not belong to him. This primary anxiety contains an indiscriminate mixture of success and failure: happiness for experiencing our own boundaries and anxiety due to the loss felt for not containing anymore inside us everything that is needed for survival. *Envy* is the anger resulting from the recognition that the other has something valuable and vital. Envy is the most denied and projected of human feelings, always fought against with magical remedies, such as herbs, protective stones, plants, potions, etc. However, protection is always sought against the envy of others, and not our own envy. Envy is considered one of the worst human feelings; both from a moral or religious perspective it is seen as a blemish or sin.

The truth is that the harshly flogged envy is an unavoidable emotion. It exists inside all human beings, to a smaller or greater extent. In spite of what I have just written, emotions are not measurable. If someone describes another person as being *very* envious, or *a bit* envious, he is quantifying and, in a way, judging. Since envy is one of the basic emotions, it is the differences in the way it is managed that will differentiate between people. Denial and projection are the most frequent forms of dealing with this fearful enemy of our self-esteem. Since neither of these two mechanisms succeeds to actually suppress envy, those who suffer from envy will refer to other people's envy as being something dangerous. And rightly so. An *envious attack* is one of the most dangerous weapons because it will always have a rationalization that justifies the attack. One of my patients told me that on the day of his graduation as a physician he invited his friends for a celebration. One of his classmates, who had to take time out from his studies due to family problems, was also present. When congratulating and embracing the graduate he told him that at this special moment he needed to make a sincere confession: he felt hurt and abandoned because the graduate did not stand by him while he was dealing with his family problems and what resulted in the temporary abandonment of his studies. 'Sincerity.' The friend told the truth, and the graduate knew that he owed his friend an apology, but the moment chosen by his friend was stimulated by a strong feeling of envy. Our lives are full of similar examples. The archetypes of *envious attacks* are Cain's crime (this will be discussed within cluster three), Judas's betrayal, or Iago, who drove Othello into a crime of jealousy. But the real and most devastating effect is related to the envious person himself. Envy is a corrosive feeling that does not allow one to be happy for someone else's success, and only generates joy at the expense of the failure of the other.

This corrosive and destructive quality of envy is closely related to the etymology of the word (in Portuguese, 'inveja'). The Latin 'invidere' means sidelong glance or squint. The Greeks used the verb 'baskainein' for a bewitched look. According to Socrates envy is a 'kind of pain', and the success of his friends turns the envious person bitter. Ventura (1998) made an etymological comparison of the words envy and cancer. Similarly to envy, the cancer or crab means something that hides. Is cancer perhaps the somatization of the corrosive envy? It could well be.

Even among the Greek gods there was a god of envy, called Ptono. But interestingly, I couldn't find his story in any of the mythology books. In Grimal's dictionary of Greek and Roman myths (1999) I found the following short reference: 'Ptono embodies envy. As with most of the demons who are only referred to by their name, Ptono does not have his own legend.' Envy moves so much within the darkness that it doesn't even have a publishable legend.

Envy is a tormenting and unbearable pain, usually a result of abandonment. A 'poisonous tongue' is often directed toward the envied person through a bitter and harmful criticism, which is socially accepted with an obliging smile. In our difficult socio-economic moments (a chronic situation in Latin America), these covert poisonous tongues usually hurt those who are successful. It is threatening because they hurt, and someone's reputation can be stained by these malicious comments. Once a rumour starts to circulate, it is impossible to stop it.

Admiration and *gratitude* are the opposites of envy; both incompatible with envy. Admiration is also often described as 'healthy envy' or 'creative envy'. The recognition that something we received is good, ennobles the giver and the receiver. For a subsequent legitimate internalization of admired positive qualities, gratitude is needed first. Acknowledging what has been received without feeling in debt also provides a right to transform it without having to be faithful to what was received. At this very moment I am adapting and transforming the ideas that I have learnt from Melanie Klein, whom I acknowledge as my first influence in psychoanalysis. However, to acknowledge doesn't mean 'to owe'. Acknowledgement sets a person free whereas debt ties him down. Acknowledging someone as my source of love, knowledge, etc., allows me to recognize him/her, without destroying the source of my growth. Unfortunately, in life there are more debts (obligations) than acknowledgements and the so much needed creativity is replaced by ritual repetition.

It is interesting to ponder for a moment what the word 'gratitude' means in different languages and different cultures. In Spanish, 'gracias' means being wishful towards the person who does something for us, with special thanks to God, as a recognition of his/her kindness. In Portuguese they say 'obrigado' that implies being obliged to someone, being in debt. In English we use 'thank you', which is closer to the Spanish meaning, or 'much obliged', referring to an obligation. In French there are also two ways to express gratitude: 'merci' and 'je suis oblige'. Thus, recognition and obligation are in collision within the various cultures.

Guilt is also steadily present in our culture, its matrix being associated to this developmental stage. While envy implies the unbearable thought that someone has something that we were denied to have, guilt is usually the opposite: we feel guilty for having something that others do not have. Guilt can be defined as a painful feeling for having committed a reprehensible act against the law or morality. It may also contain undesirable feelings or thoughts that are not compatible with the moral values that are in effect. Aguinis (1996) proposes a reconsideration of guilt as something positive that may help avoid massacres and injustices: 'I know that there is no mercy for guilt, and that a great deal of guilt is unbearable. But I would like to warn that the complete absence of guilt leads us to villainy.' Lately however, society has found certain ways to suppress guilt. Those who have power (any kind of power) tend to ignore guilt and its punishment as well; they comfortably rob and cheat. Witnessing bribery, unpunished murder, and defalcation committed by politicians and those with economic power have become part of the public ideal. The established law seems to be that if one has power one doesn't need to obey the rules. It is only a matter of waiting for the right opportunity to misuse power. Nevertheless, guilt still has a corrective influence. Thanks to guilt, humans have abandoned cannibalism and the primitive horde has adapted certain rules in order to enable survival. Thus, prohibitions and moral rules also emerge from guilt.

In front of boundaries guilt becomes an alarm signal, indicating the barrier that marks what is allowed. The problem is at the boundary of the territory. Repression serves the function of establishing allowed or forbidden territories. How and why is a territory demarcated? When something is prohibited and action is repressed, there still remains a verge to assume the desire or the impulse and to avoid carrying out this impulse as it would be against the supposedly desirable. But the feeling itself may be intolerable, erasing it from our awareness. This can go even further, suppressing the impulse, with the subsequent loss of energy.

Our Judaic-Christian culture is based more on guilt than responsibility. By responsibility I mean someone who responds and assumes. And this is a fundamental difference. It is like not committing a crime for the fear of punishment, or not committing it because of a deep conviction that it would be an erroneous action. In our everyday life, instead of understanding the established norms, infants learn much more based on the guilt–punishment dyad. 'Don't do this or that, because I will punish you, or I won't love you anymore, or I will go away and not come back, etc.' Through the fear of punishment and the lack of the understanding of rules, a guilt–punishment equation is consolidated.

It is well known that guilt has a dominating power. The anecdote of the Jewish mother, who dominates her children and her environment with suffering, is a genuine caricature of everyday scenes. Suffering becomes an internalized value, especially within the feminine universe, through the stereotypes that men cause suffering while women suffer and control through their suffering. Pain seems to be a power factor and therefore it becomes valued. These are games generated by guilt, which lose their meaning as soon as either of the partners (regardless of their gender) gains the right to develop his/her potential. Responsibility is extremely important and healthy; it means the ability to respond. Both partners assume their own responsibilities within the boundaries demarcating their co-existence.

The ideal of the Ego will be structured slowly, through internalized habits and customs. The behaviour of the infant will be defined through the approvals and disapprovals of his parents regarding what is good and bad. Before the development of the infant's own value-system, kind or strict gestures are the signals that will order his life. Guilt helps to distinguish between good and bad; however, it may happen that during the stage of differentiation between the Ego and non-Ego the internalization of these elements may become associated with the feeling of having hurt someone.

Guilt is liable to be manipulated in two fundamental ways: in a conflict situation one may assume being guilty of something until its opposite is proven; or, it may be presumed that the other is guilty. These two positions are clearly recognizable in certain people wearing the 'What did I do?' expression on their face in front of others who always seem to ask 'What did you do?' Those who belong to the 'what did I do?' group generally tend to make connections easier and more readily allow others to approach them; those belonging to the accusatory 'what did you do?' group on the other hand, tend to keep more distance. It is clear that in front of an unforeseen situation, these people will not be able to ask 'what happened?' instead of the 'what did I do?' or 'what did you do?'

Shame is another form of precocious anxiety. Predominant within the Japanese culture, it is often mistaken for guilt. The Portuguese 'vergonha' (shame) comes from the Latin 'verecundia' signifying a mood disturbance, often with a blush caused by a mistake or a disgraceful and humiliating act of oneself or somebody else. The etymology also reveals that it is a truth ('vere') that became visible and apparent ('cundere'). Shame is the sister of modesty, which was an eminently feminine virtue in the past, causing suffering for men. Blushing is a physiological reaction that becomes apparent. In contrast with guilt, when we suppose that someone has made a mistake, shame appears to reveal the true feelings of a person. For those who experience shame as a predominant feeling, the discomfort results from being revealed. They are sensitive, or in other words, stimuli are felt very intensely by them.

Shame's kinship with guilt is established through the presence of an Ego ideal that will allow certain feelings, and reject others. The expression 'shameless' makes it clear that shame was considered a virtue. However, those who often feel shame know that it is not a virtue but a great suffering. Japanese people have a profound sense of shame and hara-kiri is a consequence of it. When the high expectations of performances cannot be met, the humiliation can become so unbearable that it may lead to suicide. Failure, humiliation and self-contempt are experiences that accompany shame.

The matrix of shame is maternal overprotection. A worried mother, who takes care of her child instead of teaching the infant to take care of himself, generates a strong feeling of vulnerability. If this is accompanied by a harsh and critical paternal attitude, we are right at the origin of shame. Exposing a wrong action before others generates a feeling of humiliation, causing shyness. The child will start to anticipate situations when he/she might be exposed. Bad teachers often expose the mistake of one or another student in front of the others and by doing this progressively block their learning. It is like a continuous fear of being 'caught in the act'. 'They have realized how I really feel and I will be revealed.' In front this fear, socialization will be obstructed, the most effective defence being withdrawal.

I feel that at this point it is important to clarify the concept of *unconscious* within the Morenian theory. Moreno does not deny the existence of the unconscious; it simply cannot be denied and it would be absurd to do so. The unconscious is one of those concepts that most strongly impregnated the culture of the twentieth century. What Moreno denies is the idea of the unconscious being connected to the instincts. In the centre of Moreno's views is spontaneity, from which perspective the human being is a potential genius, and not a being who is primarily dominated by the instincts of life and death. There is no doubt, however, that genetic transmission is involved in the characteristics that form the human being. The collective unconscious is one of them, consisting of those aspects of the human being that form the baggage with which he arrives in the world. We can state with certainty that there is some sort of psychological instance that stores information. Information considered useless and therefore discarded, as well as perturbing information condemned to be forgotten, will remain stored, but once their symbolic representation is removed, they cannot be evoked.

There is another metaphor that I found useful to better understand the concept of unconscious. According to this metaphor, the unconscious is like a phrase from which many of the words have been lost and what is left is all disorganized. The elements are there but in order to understand them they need to be reorganized. This is the aim of a therapeutic process.

The ability to go through moments of pain, sorrow or frustration will depend on the internalization of the emotions and anxieties and their specific repertoires. The *internal mother* fulfils the function that will allow the going through situations of loss without disruption. The so-called *tolerance of pain* is the ability to elaborate and overcome these moments. By pain I mean feelings of guilt, shame, anxiety or fear. That is, situations primarily experienced within the 'internal' realm will tend to repeat themselves in the 'intra-personal' realm, modified by the soma (stimulus and response). Memories will result from this amalgam, in which responses play a preponderant role.

Previously (Bustos 1990) I wrote about the common origins of anxiety and spontaneity as regarding their philogenetic and ontogenetic aspects, these being phases of the same process. Here I would like to further extend the concept with the origins of *aggression*. In its primordial origin, aggression also constitutes an undifferentiated whole that can be defined as a vital ability to react to stimuli. At the beginning of life, anxiety, spontaneity and aggression converge. If positively stimulated, the infant relaxes and a smile of pleasure emerges. In case of a negative stimulus the infant will react with displeasure that will manifest itself in crying. Stimuli can be external or internal, such as hunger or any outside situation that will alter the infant's state of nirvana. In front of these stimuli the infant shows gestures of resistance by kicking and thudding without any specific direction (since his motor coordination hasn't developed yet), but with a very explicit meaning, as if he would be saying: 'I don't want this' or 'I don't like that.' In other words, aggression is basically always resistance. Anxiety is also established as a resistance that presages danger. Spontaneity (originating from within) is the quality that accompanies this action. Adequacy is an ego function that will incorporate the values that are in force within the environment.

Aggression is a necessary defence, representing an adaptive reaction in front of the attacks from the environment. But the environment is not the only trigger for these adaptive reactions. A healthy adaptive reaction can also occur in response to internal stimuli, as envy or jealousy. If, during the first phases of development, frustration persists, this will be incorporated as a constituent part of the Ego. The tension resulting from it will need to be released in order to re-establish the internal equilibrium. Finding harmony between his impulses and the rules is a fundamental struggle of the human being. Aggressive impulses without any filtering constitute psychopathy, while their complete repression will lead to depression; these two being the extreme poles of expressing aggression.

It is important to identify how aggression, envy, jealousy and rivalry will manifest themselves within the three clusters. Within the passive, dependent and incorporative first cluster, aggression usually manifests itself in the form of abandonment, leaving the other suffering from the lack of affection and sympathy. I make you feel that you need me and then I leave you alone; I abandon you. My absence is like the lack of food: it will make you powerless, or it may make you feel that you cannot live without me and so you won't be able to free yourself from me. Another form in which aggression may be manifested is mordancy, criticism or complaint. This type of aggressor never seems to be responsible for the damage he causes and he never has the intention to hurt; however, his pricks are clearly felt by their receiver. These aggressions are never overt and the aggressor usually finds thousands of rationalizations in order to justify them. However, these are only a veil for concealing the power of aggression. Sensitive persons may quickly become susceptible, and – similarly to the apparently harmless sea urchin – they may develop spikes in front of aggressors. Another image that frequently emerges during internal psychodrama sessions is that of an octopus. If someone gets too close to it he can end up caught in its tentacles. Tenderness and kindness may turn into powerful weapons.

Another form of behaviour that aggressors may take is believing that they have certain rights that others don't. The interlocutor is put in such a place where he always has to attend to his peremptory needs; however, it seems that he can never get enough. He is insatiable. The world seems to be eternally indebted to him. Or, in a reactive version, he will create the image of someone who never asks for anything. We need to remember that asking for something always opens the possibility to respond or not to respond to this need, and the person who apparently doesn't ask for anything, is actually demanding. Thus there is a chance that his needs will be seen as selfish.

We also need to take into consideration the tolerance of the other for accepting aggression (generally the partner within a couple). Every relationship has moments of frustration. Being able to tolerate these situations is essential in order not to get stuck in them (thus creating a conflict). In order to build up an adult relationship, it is fundamental to be able to digest – without disastrous responses – the aggression of the other, even when this aggression is unjustified. However, overprotected people may have the feeling that they cannot tolerate being told something violent or hard. They did not learn to defend themselves and they get depressed facing someone who does not act like a mother; they will develop a protective shield in front of the dangers of life.

Social preconditions already appear within this developmental phase. It is generally accepted that girls sojourn longer within this phase than boys. Fragility is still an acceptable characteristic for a woman. Men carry the myth of strength; they are always the ones needed, and never the ones in need. Men's self-esteem is related to the image of the provider. It seems that their message to the world is: 'I have everything to attend the needs of everybody, especially the needs of women.' Their need for contact is often disguised in sexuality: it is acceptable for the masculine self-esteem to desire sexual relationships. The more he wants them, the higher his social prestige rises. The same isn't true however for the needs of contention and tenderness, because these are considered as mainly feminine attributes. In the same way, it is more acceptable for women to confess their need for affection and company, but they must be more careful about their sexual desires in order to avoid criticism. Men and women actually have the same needs, but their relationship with these needs depends on socio-familiar conditions that still have not changed as radically as one may think.

As regarding the *therapist role* within the dynamics of cluster one, we can say that every therapeutic process happens through a succession of different moments. A hurt, deeply wounded or vulnerable patient will require a *maternal function* from the therapist. Pain can be only overcome if it has been contained first. This means that the main therapeutic dynamics are related to *holding*. Understanding and appreciative holding is most important, regardless of any other operation carried out verbally or dramatically.

Cluster two: paternal cluster

The infant slowly matures both psychologically and biologically. He sits up, experiences the strength of his legs, he reaches out for objects. He starts to master the inanimate objects, from which he learns to differentiate himself. His ability starts to manifest itself ('I can') and at the same time a new character differentiates itself from the mother: the father or the person who fulfils the *paternal function*.

Until now the role of the infant was based on the central functions of being fed, nourished and cared for (mother–child role); this will now be further expanded through a gradual conquest of autonomy, needing an auxiliary ego to teach him stand on his own feet (grounding). The complementary equation is now father–child.

Together with the action, norms also appear that will guide and direct the movement. Every norm represents a boundary for the action as well as a capacity for control. The rudimentary concepts of approval and disapproval appear. 'Don't touch the power switch'; 'You can stroke your mother but don't hit her'. As I mentioned before, the rules learned at this stage have the power of irrefutable myths, since the infant's psyche is not developed enough to have a critical ability that would filter the messages.

The transition from cluster one to cluster two is gradual and progressive and is essential for the maturation of the infant. If the first developmental phase has happened without major anxieties and the infant's rhythm of development has been respected without delaying or accelerating it, than the transition from the state of complete dependency to the gradual conquest of autonomy will happen naturally and will be experienced with spontaneity. If this natural process is disturbed, anxiety will cause a rupture and the infant's development will be delayed. This transition period coincides with the beginning of progressive discrimination between objects and persons, fantasy and reality, the Ego and non-Ego. If in cluster one the individual learns to accept his needs, the transition to cluster two will be achieved through the ability to learn to recognize, name and manage these needs.

A core sociometric concept also arises here: relationship by *criteria*. In sociometry, the sociometric criterion is the motive of choices. Someone is chosen for a specific reason. During the initial phase of life, the infant chooses his mother in all criteria because he is not distinguished from her. All of his needs are directed towards one person. Gradual growth however, will allow the infant to discriminate between his different needs, thus permitting an *alternative*. The first alternative is the father; it is possible to choose him. Thus the ability of relating to different persons (based on different criteria) develops. According to Moreno, this diversity of criteria is a healthy measure. Being able to have friends with different affinities, gives a great degree of freedom to our relationships. The ideal of finding a single person, who would fulfil all the criteria, becomes a fantasy that is at the same time desired and feared.

Both clusters one and two consist of asymmetric relationships. Both the mother–child and the father–child relationship involve two unequal roles with different responsibilities; indicating that one of the roles is dependent on and subordinated to the other. Mother and father have an active role; they respond to the biologically conditioned needs of the infant. There is no possibility of choice. More fortunate infants arrive into the world within the union of two people who chose each other and want to have a child as part of their personal achievement and their common project. Thus the conditions for a satisfactory and harmonious development are given and these will help the infant through the struggles of life.

Unfortunately though, many human beings don't have the necessary conditions to pass through these phases in a desirable way: thousands of babies are abandoned, malnourished and neglected. As a result of the precarious conditions offered by the Third World, a large number of babies live in indigence, without even having their primary needs satisfied. Character-pathologic hostility leads to the conclusion: 'Life is like this, and I am like this' – it becomes hatred that only wants to destroy in order not to be destroyed. Street children who beg, steal or vandalize, only to insult those who have what life has denied from them, represent the ignominious shame of lack and abandonment of those who had the basic conditions for their survival, but punish the less fortunate others. The defensive indifference with which we face abandonment generates a great 'mother' of social abandonment. Abandonment is not just simply an individual attitude; it becomes even crueller on a bigger social scale. 'Life is cruel and indifferent' is not just a subjective interpretation: it is the truth. This explains why the recovery of someone subjected to this abandonment is so difficult and improbable. The ability to create and dream about something better depends on the possibility of creating a memory register with a more positive reference. The fight for something desired is replaced by the invisible war against what had denied the individual's primary right for care. In spite of all this, there are people who survive emotionally thanks, probably, to genetic information that allows them to fight instead of destroying the society that insulted them.

Since the first two clusters are defined by asymmetry (indicating a person's responsibility for a helpless other), no-one in the Third World can be uninvolved in the profound social injustice in which we live, even if on an individual level some people are more favoured due to their privileged social situation. We are still all involved in what happens around us. The social guilt in front of those who don't have is part of our identity. The differences lie in what we decide to do with this situation. We can choose to deny these facts and to submerge them in indifference; or we can sooth them through donations and charity; or we can channel them through religion that forgives our sins; or we can assume the role of responsible parents, fighting with all possible resources for the inclusion of the outcast children of the Third World.

The exercise of *authority* in our shaken society depends on what was learnt in the paternal cluster. Authority can be practised through a healthy role of authority, or – on the contrary – it can be denied or applied in a distorted manner. In a previous publication (Bustos, 1992) I wrote about Adolf Hitler and the paradigm of the cruellest authoritarianism. In *Mein Kampf* he describes a scene in which he was sat on the floor drawing with great pleasure, dreaming about becoming an architect or a painter. Hitler was five or six years old at the time. His father enters the room and the boy tells him about his dream. The father replies: 'Only over my dead body.' We can imagine that this comment froze and mutilated the boy's dream. The 'corpse' had multiplied through the great number of victims of the Second World War; victims as innocent as the boy was at the time. It is likely that military dictators like Videla, Galtieri, Pinochet, etc. had had similar experiences.

The other extreme is the complete lack of authority (I don't mean here political or leadership authority). I am referring to the authority that is required to take everyday decisions throughout life. In order to know what we want, to understand our needs, and to seek what we need, the power to exercise authority is indispensable. The lack of authority is characteristic of insecure people, who seem to walk through life without purpose.

Another aspect related to cluster two is the development of the *leader* role. What makes someone become a leader? 'To lead' means to guide, to show the way. This requires initiative and the ability to generate confidence. A successful completion of cluster one will result in the person's confidence in his ability to be loved. He will know and will anticipate that people like him. As mentioned before, this self-confidence radiates a magnetism called charisma. If this self-confidence is further expanded by the company of a guide (the father), and a positive identification with the father (through the later role reversal), the individual may become a good guide for others. However, leadership may develop in another – a reactive – way.

While the predominant basic anxieties of cluster one were *envy* and *voracity*, cluster two is characterized by *jealousy*. Jealousy is defined as mental restlessness produced by the suspicion or fear of rivalry related to love or any other aspiration. Here again we are confronted with the ambiguity of the language. The words 'zêlo' and 'ciúme' (jealousy in Portuguese) have their origin in the Latin 'zelus', meaning to guard or to protect something that we own. It unites the concepts of love and possession. It is probably due to this that we admit jealousy more naturally than the reviled envy. 'I do not want to destroy what I don't have; I want it for myself' – says a jealous person.

Let us return to our friend Othello. A warrior and leader, he is envied for his strength and courage by Iago. He is clearly jealous about the ineffable Desdemona. The moment when Othello's insecurity of his possession turns into murderous fury marks the impossibility of his including vulnerability as an integral part of the courageous warrior. His lover should eternally belong to him, even if the price for this is her death. He prefers a murderous and heroic act to the mere thought of his vulnerability. Once again it is important to stress that this is not a question of the intensity of jealousy, but the way the person behaves when he feels jealous.

Synthesizing these two dynamics we could say that when cluster one predominates (and there is an absence of cluster two), the individual tends to cry instead of fighting; in the opposite case – when cluster two predominates over cluster one – the individual will fight instead of crying. Crying cannot replace fighting and fighting cannot replace crying; crying emerges from pain and sadness, while fighting from strength and the need to conquer. When these two conditions are confronted within a relationship, the outcome is a clash between the two individuals, since it is terrible to find opposition when consolation is needed, and vice versa.

Let us now see how *aggression* is dealt with in cluster two. Since it is defined through autonomy, this type of aggression is characterized by control, dominance and the tendency to establish submissive relationships.

Violence is always one of the possibilities. Physical assault, sexual abuse and violent crime are forms of aggression that belong to the paternal cluster. In its more attenuated form aggression manifests itself in persons who dictate rules and norms. They would frequently say: 'What we have to do is…', placing the other in a position of not knowing and not being able. And as long as the other submits and accepts, everything works fine. However, if the other tries to get out of this submissive position, the kindness may turn into fury. These are usually good husbands of submissive and dependant women; they are good, but at times rigid, fathers to small children.

We saw that physical violence is quite natural for people whose main wounds are related to cluster two. For quite some time it was an accepted cultural rule that 'People learn through sweating blood.' The problem with this method is that what we learn gets impregnated with the 'blood that we sweat' through this learning process. Although disapproved of, it was socially accepted that fathers and teachers physically punish their children and students. Ruling through fear and the misuse of power is a form of aggression in which identification is blocked: one can obey and respect it, but will not identify with it in a positive manner. Someone who feels secure doesn't need to use violence. This can also be observed in the behaviour of dogs. They mark their territory with urine and they only growl when somebody invades this territory. If the warning is disregarded, they attack. People who growl all the time are actually demonstrating their weakness and lack of security.

In cluster two the *role of the therapist* consists in helping the client in those moments when he needs support and affirmation (grounding). The aim is to stimulate the person's ability to fight for his goals and beliefs.

Both cluster one and two represent the cradle of *functions* that during adulthood become constituent parts of other roles. To receive (cluster one) and to give (cluster two) are fundamental functions for the dynamics of the human being. Cluster one represents the ability to say 'yes', while cluster two the ability to say 'no'. The roles of the student, patient, client, spectator, etc. are centred in the dynamics that require knowing how to receive; these are part of cluster one, their matrix being the mother–child role. The roles of the teacher, instructor, doctor and therapist on the other hand, are born out of the matrix of cluster two, with the central axis of the father–child role.

While the ability to create and generate action and ideas is related to the maternal experiences, the ability to channel and give them form is a function of cluster two. The norm that was experienced as the source of security should generate attachment. The ability to order the thoughts and actions and to give form to the contents is also the result of this learning phase. The father represents order and boundaries; therefore there is always a certain degree of aggression involved in a relationship when we say 'no'. This powerful figure who restricts omnipotence can be characterized as directing the action, which may be experienced as an amplification of the world, or as a mutilation. The rule itself should be differentiated from the agent who conveys it.

The possibility of a person identifying with the law is born within this context. Laws are formulated to protect life. Living in an organized community depends on the ability to fulfil and comply with the agreements that represent public welfare. Neglecting the responsibility of following the law leads to social chaos, endangering the survival of a country. What happens to the Latin American people, who keep infringing the law? The commanding father who created the laws has repeatedly betrayed and abandoned us. He started to use the power for his own benefit, and made us distrust the inefficient passivity. How many times did we hear the phrase: 'He is a swindler, but at least he does something' – a false, dangerous and immoral point of view. Citizenship will form within these parameters, impregnating a community that has a desire for positive action to rescue the rights of people. Social depression clearly refers to this state of things. Within this social situation, the father as a mediator in society becomes doubly important, for he can reinforce or reduce the lack of protection resulting from a hostile social environment.

We should also take into consideration another aspect of the parental influence during the first phases of development: namely, the relationship between the father and the mother. Parents form a functional unit, their relationship representing a third, seemingly invisible, but fundamental entity. Similarly to chemical elements that, when combined, give birth to a new and distinct element, the relationship of the parents will also produce new entities. Hydrogen and chlorine on their own are not the same thing as the hydrochloric acid which results from their reaction. I denominated this third element (the parental relationship) the 'third parent'. When the parental relationship reflects agreement and coherence, the child will receive messages that will help him grow. On the other hand, when the parents' relationship is disharmonic, the child will suffer from the contradictions or the annulment of the received messages. Both in marital as well as family therapy I often resort to the concretization of the relationship as a way of acknowledging the 'third parent'.

Cluster three: fraternal cluster

In the sequence of development, the infant has already learnt to walk and to pursue what he wants with the assistance of his auxiliary egos: the mother and father. This assistance indicates protective asymmetry. At this moment however, other beings appear, with whom the child will share – in one way or another – his social atom: siblings, friends, cousins, other children. Until now, in his moments of rage he attacked his parents, who reproved and complaisantly taught him not to do that. Now however, there are new beings around that react differently: when attacked, they return the blow without thinking; they are equals. *Symmetry* generates the majority of roles performed in adulthood. The complementary equals are the siblings.

In clusters one and two we didn't have a distinct name for the relationships; these relationships were simply indicated by isolated roles. They are asymmetric and should be named separately. The same is true for all relationships of unequal responsibility: teacher–student, doctor– patient, etc. Based on the fraternal relationship, all other relationships implying symmetry will have a distinct name: friends, brothers, partners, companions, colleagues, lovers, etc. (Bustos 1979).

Most of the adult roles develop within this cluster. Clearly, the two previous experiences are fundamental in order to go maturely through the fraternal cluster. In order to learn to share, the child first needs to be supported (contained) and he needs to gain confidence. *Holding* gives way to *grounding*, following which *sharing* appears; thus the three main dynamics of the human being are formed.

Learning to share and abandoning the fantasy of 'everything belongs to me' is always painful, and it implies giving up the omnipotence and tyranny that reined the first evolutionary stages. 'May the brothers be united' – said Martin Fierro (in a book by the Argentine José Hernandez). However, the first mythical image regarding brothers comes from the story of Cain and Abel, in which one destroys the other out of jealousy and envy. But this is not a primary emotion; it is only a representation of the murder that springs from God's favouritism (God being a metaphor for father–mother), who praises the presents of Abel and despises Cain's. It is this attitude of God that inflicts Cain's hatred, who – instead of confronting God's injustice – directs his murderous aggression against his brother. As always, human emotions are not *chemically pure*. Cain is envious as well as jealous. The ultimate motive for the fraternal crime is envy. As mentioned earlier on, the equation of envy is *to destroy the person who has something desired*. *Rivalry* urges one *to block the path of the rival in order to defeat him*. The first emotion is more primary and destructive; the second consists in destroying in order to win.

Aguinis (1999) mentions a theory according to which Cain was actually a child born from Eve's adultery with a demon; his descendants gave origin to the Black, Latin, Oriental, Hispanic and Jewish races. From Abel, legitimate son of Adam and Eve, originates the pure Arian race, rightful inheritors of the Earth. From this perspective, the myth of Cain and Abel may explain prejudices. This seemingly absurd theory is at the basis of religious fundamentalism, with which some of the most horrendous crimes are justified (such as the holocaust). It also kills many birds with only one stone: it considers women (due to their disobedience and innate impurity) the cause of all bad; and, all non-Arian to be usurpers of the Kingdom of God. In another version of this story, Lilith is considered to be the mother of all impure and demonic non-Arian beings, who usurp the legitimate place of Adam's and Eve's pure children.

Relationships that result from symmetry are characterized by three different dynamics: *sharing, competition* and *rivalry*. Sharing is the most desirable, but also the most difficult to achieve within our society. Like an omnipotent and unjust God, our society confronts people, favouring some to the disadvantage of others. Dominant races murder the more unfortunate ones, who don't even have the slightest chance for survival. Those who have a privileged economic situation ignore and murder the innocent 'Abels', play with the life of human beings, and justifying their actions through their own power. Under these circumstances it is difficult to share (that is, to become 'us' without predominance).

Sharing requires the desire to contribute (with what we have) to the public well-being. Moreno wrote about sharing with passion, both as a *desideratum* of human communication, and as the third phase of the psychodrama session. In the first Spanish and Portuguese psychodrama publications this third phase was called the phase of 'comments or analysis'; thus the original meaning, as formulated by Moreno, became distorted. According to Moreno, within the phase of sharing each group member should talk about himself, and not about the protagonist. This also refers to the director, who is required to abandon his position of therapist and share his personal experiences evoked by the dramatization from a symmetrical position. The phase of sharing is not aimed at discussing the protagonist, or at analysing his behaviour; the objective is to enable everyone to share their own experiences and, through these shared experiences, to reach new group knowledge. The power of asymmetry always becomes hierarchical with one dominating over the other; as we saw above, during the first phases of development this is necessary for survival. So power is necessary, but if it is maintained longer than necessary, it will become unhealthy. This power will try to perpetuate and impose itself, for itself. It may lead to fraternal confrontation, or to an amorous dependency that imprisons and controls. The choice disappears and the healthy desire to be with the other turns into the destructive 'I cannot live without you', that may even become an ideal of love. Cluster three requires from us a dangerous and responsible ability to make permanent choices. To be able to choose and to be chosen, are mature and responsible forms of establishing relationships. In the absence of this option, a (overtly or covertly) hostile relationship appears.

Situations when we share are rare, but everybody is familiar with the feeling of fulfilment achieved through joint action where each one contributes something of his own, without questioning how much the others have contributed. On a social level, Fidel Castro's proposal follows this ideal: everyone contributes with his best in order to achieve a goal. However, the human being is not so altruistic; his narcissistic needs are just as important as his need to participate in a common project. When looking at various proposals, North-Americans very naturally ask: 'What do I gain from this?' We don't feel so much at ease with this tranquillity of individualism, which opposes the idealized detachment. Within our ideal of the Ego (I) we have the archetype of Christ, who assumed neither the role of the father nor that of the mother; instead, he assumed the role of the brother, who gave everything to his brethren. This is total detachment, an indifference (unconcern) towards our personal needs in exchange for the common welfare; a kind of anti-Cain, who puts his brother in the first place. Setting this Christian ideal (dominating most of the western world, with millions of followers) against the 'What do I gain from this?', would lead to a sinister result.

The development of this desirable ability to *share* becomes hampered in our individualistic society, where our value is measured by what we earn. Within this society self-esteem is based on personal earnings. Maybe in the developed countries it is possible to survive with this attitude; here in the Third World, is not. Competition is stimulated from early childhood (at school, in sports, etc.) with the following basic value being added to it: being good at something and using your potential is not important; what is important is to be *better than others* – thus, competition will prevail over sharing. While, in the archetype of Christ the social ideal is idealized, competition – promoting exactly the opposite – is always accompanied by guilt and dissociation: on Sundays I go to church to praise the Lord, and later I do exactly the opposite. Happiness (meaning to be in peace with oneself) cannot be achieved this way. Our society offers alcohol, nicotine and drugs (poisonous-remedies) as commercial antidotes for this strong dissociation.

Competition is a dynamic that has always existed in the explicit form of championships, sports, etc. The Olympic Games are an eloquent proof of this. Competition has always been present within the human race.

Nowadays however, the disgusting amounts of money that are at stake, lead to the objective of 'getting to the top at any price'.

This premise of 'at any price', takes us to the third dynamic of cluster three: *rivalry*. If one cannot win by applying one's maximum potential, one will try to obstruct the triumph of the other. When confronted with the fear of losing, one would impede or obstruct the path of the other, placing obstacles in front of his adversary. This can also be observed during election campaigns. When in a favourable position candidates talk about their programme, and their conditions to carry this out. This is fair play. However, when another candidate also gains a favourable position, details of this adversary's private life start to be revealed, stressing those aspects that may denigrate him in front of the electors. This has always happened in a more or less intense way. But today it takes place in a clear and evident manner — naturally. We don't rebel against those who apply these resources; we just simply listen to what they want to say. Events from the candidate's adolescence, their private and internal characteristics are revealed and used as lawful resources. If this was an attitude that stayed within the ring of dirty political fights, it would simply be disapproved of, and nothing else. But as it happens, these public figures represent images that we identify with: by doing what they do, they legitimize everyone to do the same in their private world. Thus, deceit and lack of scruples become part of the Ego ideal as being permitted.

Negotiation is essential within the relationships of cluster three. Agreements are born out of symmetrical relationships in which one is ready to give up something in order to gain something else. The initial passion and dreams of marital relationships give the illusion of being one again, eternally indivisible and inseparable. During this initial phase negotiation is not necessary; there is no rivalry or envy. The partners form a unit. Projective identification protects from comparisons. Time however, painfully annihilates this illusion. Similarly to the end of the matrix of undifferentiated all-identity, the other separates, removing and carrying with him or herself all his or her riches, leaving behind loss, pain, aggression and resentment. In order to maintain the relationship, negotiation is necessary. How is this possible, when they used to want the same things, and used to have the same preferences? Actually, this wasn't so. 'I don't like football, I prefer cinema; I get bored in the theatre; television is for idiots.' These are agreements and negotiations in which the Ego (I) impetuously fights against the We. This fighting for power and control may become exhausting at times.

Working towards the *we* is a characteristic of cluster three. Cluster one already contains this *we* in a rudimentary form, which will be accentuated in cluster two. However, in both cases the asymmetry of the relationship ensures that the rules are established by one of the roles (mother and/or father). These rules are in fact imposed, which is good considering that the infant does not know how to alter them. In cluster three however, fighting is established, teaching the child to negotiate, to give in, and to progress. Submission ensures a relationship that is maintained only by control.

Aggression as a modality of cluster three usually manifests itself in the form of fights, clashes and arguments. This type of person seems to say: 'I am right, no matter what.' They spend a lot of time challenging imaginary opponents or creating opponents within their close relationships. They always seem to have a rival or an opponent around. 'Yes, but...' seems to be their most frequent phrase.

Some time ago society approved of parents who beat their children, considering that this was 'educational'. This approach actually legitimized and justified rivalry at 'any price'. It doesn't matter how; what is important is to win. A few years ago an ice-skater asked some friends to break her rival's leg in order to win a competition. Destroy in order to win. This case was published in the papers, together with the case of a girl who cut the face of her beautiful friend, or the case of fearsome football supporters chanting 'together we'll destroy' instead of 'together we'll win'. The climate of high tension reigning companies is worrying but also illustrative. A nice colleague with whom we get along may turn into a despicable enemy, at the sign of us being 'off guard'. Cains and Abels facing an almighty God, who doesn't share his favours, but confronts and profits from confrontations.

This type of aggression is dangerous, because there is no-one in the relationship who would assume (at least theoretically) responsibility, as it was the case in clusters one and two. This dynamic is reigned by the idea of 'everyone for himself'. This frenzy may lead to chaos. A resource often used in order to handle this destructiveness is to create an easily identifiable enemy. 'Together we are strong.' However, this togetherness may become difficult in front of the various manifestations of misery and abandonment. In this case, we can resort to locate the enemy: Manchester United vs. Arsenal, blacks vs. whites, Jews vs. Christians, etc. There will always be a secure and identifiable place for the enemy that will legitimize (and make more understandable) this aggression reigning human beings as a reformulation of the primitive hordes.

The *role of the therapist* within cluster three consists in the therapist's ability to make available his own experiences (that are similar to those of the client) in a grown-up experiential interchange. However, it isn't always appropriate to tell these experiences; for some patients it may be important to preserve their mythical depositions and this should be respected. Transference is always involved and experiences shared within transferential situations may become distorted, generating unnecessary tensions.

Beyond sharing experiences, an adult-to-adult understanding is also present here, an attitude that generates a strongly reparative relationship. 'I know how you feel, because I have also been there.' At times it is important to specify the experiences, always keeping in mind that although these are fraternally shared, therapy is based on an asymmetric relationship. And this is good, since the responsibilities of one and the other are different. If we mystify, pretending that non-existing symmetries are present between patient and therapist, we only produce a fallacy, a mere illusion of a relationship that will not allow the flow of truth, which is necessary in order to understand the soul of a suffering person.

Final considerations

My intention within this chapter was to reflect on the past ten years of my work as a psychotherapist and it is a privilege to know that my colleagues consider my thoughts useful for their clinical work. My starting point was the relationship as a unique, tangible and concrete aspect allowing me to penetrate the inner world with its subjectivity. However, when converted into thoughts through the relentless Aristotelian logic, feelings and sensations become mutilated and limited. And this is even more so when trying to translate them into written language. Written words never reflect exactly what one is trying to say.

Cybernetics has created a new form of expression. Computers not only invaded markets, but also subjectivity. There is a vertiginous change around us that we can only observe with surprise. Youngsters incorporate these changes while us 'oldies' painfully recognize that we are left aside. As we saw, this may become the source of envy; an envy that may be painfully accepted or converted into inexorable criticism. Since the beginnings of the world, the generations who had lost their vigour and power, always made apocalyptic predictions concerning the changes of which they are not part anymore. As time goes by, or as we go through time, we change from being protagonists to being audience; as audience we can assist what is happening or we may fight for protagonism through a destructive criticism. As observers, we can participate with our experience, as long as our pride will allow us. What we cannot do however, is to ignore the changes leading to new theories, because this is what is going to change the way subjectivity is formed. If we want to continue acting in the theatre of life, we have to be able to reformulate our concepts and beliefs. Moreno predicted that only those who are spontaneous will survive in the new millennium. Now, at the beginning of the new millennium we can say that only through our capacity to constantly re-create our universe will we be able to stay in touch with the deep sense of life.

Note

1 Originally published under the title: 'As marcas da vida: A teoria dos clusters'. In D.M. Bustos (2001) *Perigo…Amor a Vista! [Danger…Love at Sight!])* Second extended edition. São Paulo: Aleph.

7

Digression around certain aspects of role theory[1]

Sergio Perazzo

I think that we psychodrama psychotherapists have been looking at the roles through the old fashioned lens of a pince-nez, and not through the more up-to-date optics of a telescope, of a magnifying glass, of a microscope or even that of the naked eye. What I am suggesting is that, even if we may not be fully skilled in the use of all these instruments, we shouldn't consider Moreno's ideas as finished and complete, but should try and look at them through a critical perspective. When examining more rigorously the role theory, Rocheblave-Spenlé (a French sociologist) has pointed out certain feeble aspects of Moreno's vision, doing this however, without devaluing his contributions and creations. Perhaps because of being a psychiatrist, Moreno did not place the deserved emphasis on the regularity of the social processes, on the institutional character of social life, and neither did he stress enough the importance of culture as well as that of social norms and values; he applied more of a micro-social perspective, exaggeratedly privileging the individual. This critique has been endorsed among us over the last few years, through the direct or indirect contributions of psychodrama authors, such as Gonçalves dos Santos or Alfredo Naffah Neto.

While on the one hand Moreno contrapositions the originality of the individual with the conformity of society (in a way denying the social determinants), on the other hand, sociologists theorizing about the roles (opposing and criticizing certain aspects of the Morenian work) did not manage to assimilate and thoroughly understand the concepts of role reversal and encounter. They interpret Moreno's well-known poem (in which he defines these concepts through the exchange of eyes) as one observing himself as an object. That is, they also apply the lens of a pince-nez.

In order to illustrate the difficulty and complexity of this issue of the role concept, let us examine some of the thoughts presented by Anibal Mezher (1980), one of the first Brazilian psychodramatists to review the subject of roles, and the first one to question the concept of psychosomatic roles[2] created by Moreno. Based on his study of role complementarity, Mezher questions the validity of this concept. According to him, in case of the 'psychosomatic roles', this complementarity – understood as interaction between people through roles and their corresponding counter-roles – is absent. What is, for example, the complementary role for that of the ingestor? – asks Mezher.[3] After a thorough and careful analysis of the various role concepts, Mezher arrives to the following definition: 'role is a specific conjunction of actions that – according to a model established by a certain society – takes place in the interaction of human beings' (Mezher 1980, p.221). His definition is based on three basic aspects that are also included in numerous other role definitions,[4] these being considered as parts of the role concept.

Based on his analysis, Mezher also considers that when it involves a relationship with an object or an animal, the denomination of role is inadequate. Thus, he questions whether a cavalryman or a sculptor can be considered as roles. Although I am aware that Mezher's paper (1980) is only a summary of his ideas and that I am picking on a small detail, I would still like to propose the following argument.

From a social perspective, the recognition of these two roles (cavalryman and sculptor) is unquestionable. In a social gathering or party for example, it is possible to introduce So-and-So, a famous sculptor, or So-and-So, a cavalryman (or knight) from Her Majesty's Guard, without this causing any surprise among the guests. (A knight perhaps would be seen as slightly strange, since we don't live in a kingdom, except the kingdom of 'King Momo', elected every February as the king of the Carnival.) Thus, the first role (the sculptor) would be recognized immediately, just as would the second (cavalryman/knight), although we would need to quickly relate this latter to the context from whence he comes (another country, obviously a monarchy), or possibly a symbolic kingdom of our own country (the Carnival). Therefore, through these roles the actual individual can be introduced, complemented by his own social identity. Regardless of the sculpture or the horse, an interrelation can occur between these roles and other human beings. The role becomes an attribute of the individual, bestowed by a consensus of society itself, while the set (conjunction) of actions specifically related to the marble or the horse represent an aggregate that precedes the relationship with the others (although these define the same role, they do not contain any interrelational elements or aspects). The sculptor and the cavalryman in this case represent a social label and are related to other roles: cavalryman-guard and, respectively, sculptor-artist.

Rocheblave-Spenlé describes a variety of real roles, an example of these being the mother role, whose definition involves a sexual quality (woman), an age-related quality (adult) and a family-related quality (wife, although this is not indispensable). The complementarity and the involvement of these qualities however, are absent or diluted in those roles that depend on the 'concatenation of time': the role of the adult man for example, occurring from the adolescent, which in its turn occurs from the child. This variable of time is also present in those roles that define the stages of a career. Moreno is often criticized for not including a dramatic denotation in his role definition – a criticism that seems questionable to me, because Moreno's intention was to amplify the role concept, both in its inter-personal and intra-personal sense. In my understanding the underlying idea of Moreno's intention to amplify the role concept is that: firstly, society can in itself supply elements to define the role, and secondly, everything that can be enacted can be converted into a dramatic role, even if it is not a social role.

Rocheblave-Spenlé has summed up the parameters (considered by various authors) that define the role in the following way:

1. On the group level – a behavioural model that applies to everyone who possesses the same *status*. This behavioural model is defined through consensus and it expresses cultural norms and values.

2. On the inter-personal level – the role consists of reciprocal forms of behaviour or behavioural models within the process of interaction that occur in response to the expectations of the other, and depend on the specific situation.

3. On the level of the personality – it represents an attitude towards the other, a social habit of the individual that is closely related to the 'deeply-routed personality', or the I. (Rocheblave-Spenlé 1969, p.145).

Comparing Rocheblave-Spenlé's above-presented parameters with that of Mezher's role definition, we can notice the different purposes of these two authors: departing from the action, Mezher moves to the interaction mediated by a social model; Rocheblave-Spenlé focuses on the conduct or behavioural model that already contains in itself the social element (even on the inter-personal level), the other (person) also being a representative of the same society, to whose expectations the individual needs to respond in a specific situation (the personality being the modeller of the way the individual will act).

This view becomes even clearer when Rochable-Spenlé arrives at his own – supposedly generic – role definition: 'role is an organized behavioural model that relates to a certain position of the individual in an interactional conjunction' (1969, p.172). My impression is that Mezher (as a psychodramatist) cannot disconnect the role concept from the context in which he studied it (that is, psychodrama), establishing between them the act– action link. Rocheblave-Spenlé (whose area of investigation is sociology) on the other hand, embodies the individual within the social situation (conjunction). It is also interesting to note the plural that Mezher uses regarding the actions ('conjunction of actions') and the singular of Rocheblave-Spenlé's 'organized behavioural model'. On the other hand, by inserting the individual into an 'interactional conjunction', Rocheblave-Spenlé pluralizes the denotation of the relationship, while Mezher uses the singular 'interaction between human beings'. The impression is that they are both saying the same thing; however, if we read more carefully between the lines, the differences between their preoccupations become obvious.

Furthermore, Rocheblave-Spenlé distinguishes the following three particular role categories:

1. Social role – here the [individual's] position becomes *status*; the behavioural model is defined by the group members through their consensus, having a functional value for this group.

2. Dramatic role – the position [of the individual] is provided by the theme of the theatrical play; the model – created by the playwright – will define the [role] play of the actor.

3. Personal role – the individual himself determines his position in relation to others, acting according to his own behavioural model that promotes the norms of inter-personal relationships.' (Rocheblave-Spenlé 1969, p. 172)

This being the case, we can say that there is a part of the role totality (in the case of the sculptor and the cavalryman represented by their relationship with the marble and the horse — that precede the individual's relationships with others) that is nothing more than one of the guidelines that mark and shape the position of the cavalryman and the sculptor and that pre-configure their behavioural model (this latter including both the function and the position); it is through this behavioural model they can be socially recognized, as a sculptor and a cavalryman.

Therefore, it does not seem difficult for me to understand the different role definitions along Moreno's work, as long as I understand him within the various dimensions of this subject. As with the personality (if developed in a perennial movement, subjected to the limitations of a particular conceptualization, which consequently becomes incomplete, since it tries to include it in a rigid system of references), the role — closely related to the personality and equally dependent on a social dynamism — cannot be delineated through fully satisfactory parameters. It was Moreno himself who wrote that because of being connected to the personality (*persona*), the role integrates private, social and cultural elements, and it can promote inter-personal changes. This statement of Moreno was also highly regarded by Rocheblave-Spenlé.

In order to further expand this reflection about role theory, let us now look at the question of the psychodramatic, or psychological, or imaginary roles.

Moving on from the world of undifferentiated sensations (characteristic of the first phase of the matrix of identity, or the 'first universe') to the bi-dimensional world (social and fantasy world) of the 'second universe' (the breach between fantasy and the experience of reality), will result in the development and performance of the social roles and of what Moreno called psychodramatic roles. In the category of psychodramatic roles Moreno included both the roles performed on the fantasy level, and those that enfold within a psychodramatic scene.

Although he acknowledges the similarities within the structure of these two forms of the psychodramatic role, José Fonseca (1980) prefers to use the term 'psychodramatic role' only for the roles performed within a psychodramatic scene, while he uses the term 'psychological' or 'fantastic' role for the former ones (that is, roles performed on the fantasy level), also including in this category roles that result from a delirant activity.

Alfredo Naffah Neto (1979) on the other hand, uses the term 'dramatic role' for roles originating in theatre; and, because with the passage from the 'first universe' to the 'second universe' the performance of the social roles tends to banish the imaginary world into a secondary level, he calls the roles that belong to this world 'imaginary roles'. Naffah Neto reserves the term 'psychodramatic role' for those roles that emerge from:

> a new synthesis between the imagination and action, between the spirit and the body; deservedly resuming the individual in its joint existence and dissolving its previous split between the social role and the private person (where the role described the action and the private person described the imagination). (Naffah Neto 1979, p.196)

In his view, the imaginary roles are dislocated from, and so not transformed into real action (dreams and reveries), while the psychodramatic roles are the concretizations in action of the imaginary roles.

Because they do not fit into his definition of social roles, when referring to these (imaginary) roles Rocheblave-Spenlé compares them to those of infantile play, including them in the category of the roles of the imagination. He observes that while social roles result in the 'performance of a role', the roles of the imagination can only become visible 'through the performance of a role'. He also mentions the term imaginary role, but uses the word 'imaginary' only as a qualitative expression, and not as a (role) classification. Thus, since it doesn't fulfil a specific function within a group, and because it is not established or defined by society, in Rocheblave-Spenlé's view this role (of the imagination) conveys to the specific categories of the dramatic role or the personal role. As we saw, Moreno's denomination of the psychodramatic role embodies in itself what Rocheblave-Spenlé calls the dramatic roles and the personal roles. Now we can understand better why Fonseca separates the psychodramatic roles into psychodramatic and psychological (or fantastic) roles; and why Naffah Neto distinguishes between dramatic, imaginary and psychodramatic roles; while Rocheblave-Spenlé, without finding an appropriate space for the roles of the imagination, places them either in the category of the dramatic roles, or in the category of personal roles, depending on their characteristics.

From the perspective of the sociologist Rocheblave-Spenlé, the definition of the dramatic role is connected to the theme of a theatre-play (as position) and to the performance of the actor, for which the playwright's script supplies the model. The definition of the personal role on the other hand, is connected to the theme of the individual (as position), having the individual's norm of action (created within the realm of the inter-personal) as its model. In my view however, this denomination ('personal role') may be misleading. Is it possible to have a role, any role, which is not personal?

In Moreno's view, within a psychodrama scene the psychodramatic role includes both, the dramatic and the personal aspect of Rocheblave-Spenlé, while outside the psychodrama scene, it coincides with the personal role. Therefore, I support the intention of Fonseca and Naffah Neto when they try to define these concepts more precisely, even though there is certain dissatisfaction regarding the terms introduced by them. For, while Fonseca reserves the word 'psychodramatic' for the roles performed within the psychodrama scene, the prefix *psycho-* still seems to suggest something more, thus intuitively getting closer to Naffah Neto's definition. When separating the psychodramatic roles into dramatic, imaginary and psychodramatic ones, Naffah Neto is more precise in his definitions.

In this sense it seems more appropriate to me to call dramatic role the role as it was defined by Rocheblave-Spenlé, the role connected to the script, containing the theme conserved by an author (that can even be the actual actor). As for the psychodramatic role, I prefer to use the redefinition introduced by Naffah Neto, that is, the imaginary role that – created by the author-actor and initiated within a psychodrama scene – spontaneously turns into real action. I believe that in the absence of a more appropriate name, preserving the term 'psychodramatic' is justified in the light of the above definition; preserving this term also seems important in order not to overload this already controversial theory with even more new concepts. For the same reason, I believe that the terms 'psychological', 'fantastic' or 'imaginary' role should also be freed from this 'jail of synonyms' and should be used in the senses given by Fonseca and Naffah Neto. In my view, using either of these three terms may be appropriate.[5] And as with Rocheblave-Spenlé's definition of the private, psychological, fantastic or imaginary roles, these would fit perfectly well into his category of the personal role (however, I still sustain my critique for the term 'personal'), that will go beyond the simply imaginary. By 'going beyond' the imaginary I mean that – since being established – these roles created by the individual will be performed in real life in relation to others. They are borrowed from the cult that surrounds certain people elevated by the divulging organs (such as arts, politics, sports, etc.) to the condition of stardom or hero, and without involving any delirium, they are at the same time within the realm of the real and the fantastic. The psychodramatic role (understood as in the psychodramatic scene) already contains elements of the dramatic as well as the personal role, constituting in itself an original category that was not considered by the sociologists.

Notes

1 Originally published under the title: 'Digressão sobre uns quantos pontos da teoria da papéis'. In S. Perazzo (1986) *Descansem em Paz os Nossos Mortos Dentro de Mim [Let Our Dead Rest in Peace inside Me]*. São Paulo: Ágora, pp.81–90, 1995.

2 The psychosomatic roles, as defined by Moreno, are the first roles to be performed by the human being, and are connected to vital functions; these are the role of the ingestor, of the defecator and the urinator.

3* Based on the concept of corporal zones and family roles, Mezher proposes to substitute the concept of psychosomatic role with the concept of *corporal zone in (inter)action*. And, in order not to get in contradiction with Moreno's postulate according to which the roles are the tangible aspects of the self (the self developing from them), Mezher further adds: 'the corporal zones are corporal areas that function in relation to the world, with an increasing experiential process of the body in relation to the world and its own components (processes that are concomitant and integrated with the individual's social experience); these zones are important factors in the consolidation of the corporal identity, a basis that is adequate for the foundation of the "ego" [self]' (Mezher 1980, p.223). Thus, according to Mezher, the psychosomatic roles can be seen as corporal zones in (inter)actions that are involved in the mother–child relationship as well as other family roles, without threatening the corporal identity of the child.

4* These three basic aspects are: interaction between humans, joint action and the subordination to a model established by society.

5* In one of his more recent books Perazzo (1994) has introduced a further refinement regarding the imaginary roles. He distinguishes between the imaginary roles encapsulated within the individual, who is unable to enact them easily (within a psychodramatic scene) due to a blockage resulting from a transference issue (he denominates these 'transferential imaginary roles'); and 'fantasy roles' (or 'non-transferential imaginary roles'), these being un-enacted imaginary roles that are not blocked by transference issues, and so can be more easily and spontaneously transformed into action within a psychodrama scene, a role-play, a spontaneous theatre session, or infantile play.

8

The protagonist and the protagonic theme[1]

Luís Falivene R. Alves

As a result of the developing psychodrama theory and technique, there is a necessity for a more in-depth study of certain elements and concepts of psychodrama. Previously established expressions, such as the 'protagonist of the group' or 'the group as protagonist', bring us to a fundamental issue: the need for a more exact conceptualization of this psychodramatic instrument – the protagonist.

Nowadays, the term protagonist is usually used to indicate the most apparent group member whose participation is prevalent within a certain psychodramatic event. Without sticking to the correct and appropriate meaning of the term, artists, sportsmen, politicians, outlaws, corrupt people or even victims have all been called protagonist. This popularization of the meaning has led to a tendency of calling protagonist both a member of the group who stands out in the group context, as well as the client in individual therapy.

From the perspective of the psychodrama methodology, this could result in certain incongruence: we start our dramatic work *taking the protagonist for granted*, for whom the text needs to be adapted; or, even worse, we start from a pre-existing script elaborated for a certain protagonist. In both cases we are invalidating the essence of the therapeutic theatre, that is, creaturgy – the dramaturgy of the moment.

When establishing the five instruments of psychodrama (stage, protagonist, director, auxiliary ego and audience), Moreno had as reference the psychodramatic method – or more specifically, the dramatic context. Within the group context, there is a division of roles: on the one hand we have the people who are interested in or require the dramatic action (the clients), and on the other hand the technical team consisting of one or more members (such as, coordinator, supervisor, therapist, co-therapist, etc.). The nomination, within the group context, of the clients and the technical team as being protagonist, audience, director or auxiliary ego, is only an anticipation of what will occur in the following phase, that is, in the dramatic context. While it is possible to make this prevision regarding the professionals (that is, we know beforehand that Dr So-and-so will be the director, and Dr So-and-so will be the auxiliary ego), we cannot say the same about the functional unit that participates in the therapy. The same is true for situations when the technical team consists of only one professional; how can we foresee which group members will be asked to act as auxiliary egos?

It further adds to this terminological confusion that we often read and hear, that in a sociodramatic situation the protagonist is the group, while actually what we want to elucidate is that the objective of such a dramatic act would be to attend to the (intra- or inter-group) demands created by the group, considering the group itself as the client. It is incorrect to call the group protagonist, especially if we consider that in many sociodramatic situations (focused on intra-group difficulties or readjustments), we use interactive and perceptive games, or sociometric investigation, in which cases there is no protagonization; protagonization only occurs when the context becomes dramatic.

Another inaccuracy is to affirm that the protagonist was the theme, mistaking it for what is called the protagonic theme.

In its wider sense, the protagonic theme is the text, script or the subject matter (plot) that is built up and developed during the psychodramatic act; this protagonic theme is expressed through the protagonist, who is responsible for its development and outcome. The protagonic theme has its premises within the social context, it is outlined within the group context, and it is developed and defined within the dramatic context. At the same time as he unveils the protagonic theme, the director also propitiates the emergence of the protagonist; this will always happen through characters (real, symbolic or metaphoric) that are exclusive of the dramatic context. This conceptual rigour is necessary in order to consider that protagonization is the actual reason or motive of psychodrama.

Before defining the protagonist further, let us first see a clinical example that will serve as a warm-up for later reflections and considerations. Let us imagine the following psychotherapeutic psychodrama session.

The protagonic theme

As he always does, the therapist goes to the waiting room of his office in order to receive the members of the therapy group, at the same time listening to the conversation that develops between them. In this case, the group members are talking about films they saw and that were nominated for the Academy Award, about the interests of the media, about the possible award winners, etc. For the psychodrama director this represents the first contact with the *protagonic theme*, that is, *to win or to lose*.

After the group members enter the therapy room, they carry on with this conversation for a while. A short silence follows, when the beginning of the therapeutic context is announced. After discussing some of the issues that the group dealt with in previous sessions, one of the group members (Daniela) talks about the possibility of her losing her job, examining the fact that she never managed to progress within her profession. Since unemployment is a general issue in the whole country, the group shows their sympathy and strong involvement with Daniela. Thus, the *protagonic theme* further develops: *winning or losing, continuing/persisting or starting again?* Since the group incites this theme, the director proposes dramatic work.

A starting scene is suggested: an encounter between Daniela and her professional role. Renata (another member of the group) is chosen to represent this professional role. However, she is reluctant and refuses to play the role: she feels sad, angry and prefers not to take part in the scene; she has just discovered that her marriage is threatened by another woman. The group's attention turns towards Renata; they want to know what happened to her, and so at this moment they lose their interest in Daniela. Daniela and the director are both on the stage, but what can be done?

As Daniela has already been nominated protagonist, does it mean that we are trapped in this decision? Do we need to try and find something to blame for the situation (such as the lack of warm-up, our precipitation, or a false protagonist)? Or, would we consider Renata's attitude as a manipulating and transferential act of her triangular situation? It could be all of this, or none of this. However, it is better to deal with the situation as psychodramatists, considering the situation as a further development of the protagonic theme: *winning or losing, continuing or starting again, competing-arguing or being excluded.*

OK, but what do we do now? Daniela and the director are on the psychodramatic stage, and the group has turned to Renata. We need to understand that we are still within the group context and did not move on to the dramatic context. The protagonist hasn't emerged yet; however, we need to respect Daniela and her warm-up for action. The director invites Renata onto the stage. Holding both of their hands, he assures his containment for both Daniela and Renata, addressing the group in the following way:

> Daniela and Renata have presented their distress in front of the possibility of losing their roles of employee and wife, respectively. Daniela and I have started our warm-up for dramatization and were also threatened to lose our roles when you started to ask questions from Renata. What we have here is a theme that belongs to all of us: the threat of losing a person, a role, a job. Questions of love touch our souls deeply, but in these various situations we are talking about the love for another, the love of the other, or even the love for ourselves. Which one of us can undertake the dramatic development of this theme? Daniela or Renata? Or maybe someone else from the group? Daniela or Renata?

With this attitude the director confirms the idea that the protagonist will be the character emerging within the dramatic context; it will not be Daniela nor Renata, but a representative of everyone who is willing to investigate the proposed issue, with the objective of transforming it.

Noticing the emotional climate of the group, Daniela says: 'I think that Renata is in more distress; if she explores her situation, it will also help me.' The group indicates their concurrence:

Director: [still addressing Daniela, preparing her return to the audience]: Just a while ago we were warming up for your scene, and now we will do the same with Renata. Would you like to suggest a scene for her? [The intention of the director with this question is to sustain the complicity between the two of them.]

Daniela: It could be a scene with Renata having a conversation with her husband about their marriage.

Renata: It could be, but this would be a scene full of jealousy, aggression and regrets for what was said. What is worst is this feeling I have, a sort of identification, a kind of confusion.

Director: So, let's start with this feeling. Are you OK Renata? Daniela? [She is already sitting in the audience.] Everything OK with the group? ... Renata, close your eyes and try to get in touch with this confusion. Let the

> sensations express themselves through your movements, voice, your words.

Since nothing occurs to Renata, the director suggests to her to be the actual confusion.

> *Director*: Confusion, I would like you to transform Renata [at this moment played by another group member] into a character.

The character of a damsel emerges (clearly influenced by the films that were discussed in the waiting room). The chosen scene is that of the young damsel having to marry a prince she doesn't love. As this scene dramatically unfolds, the sense of confusion reappears in the confrontation of the damsel with three other characters: a monarch (the father), reminding her of the nobility of this gesture; a pious mother, talking about the value of sacrifice; and a peasant girl beckoning the beauty of freedom and passion. Through the use of psychodramatic techniques the conflict between mother/sacrifice and peasant girl/freedom is intensified. The apex is reached when the mother reveals that after the nearly fatal birth of her daughter, she made a pledge: she would bring up her daughter to save the people and the nation. As an adult, the young damsel was afraid that if she did not follow her destiny (that is, marry the prince, and save her people), she would die. Thus, the protagonic theme is further developed: *winning or losing, continuing or starting again, competing/ arguing or being excluded, to live or to die*. The damsel needs to choose between a life that she has been offered and a free life; conservation and creativity; life and death. Through the use of the mirror technique, she gains a decisive perception: the real death would be accepting the pre-determined life. The damsel decides to renounce the crown and to live free. Now, however, she feels very lonely; while before she could rely on those who predisposed her life, now she doesn't have anyone. One of the auxiliary egos offers her help: the young peasant girl extends her arms towards the damsel. The director asks if anybody else wants to accompany her, and the whole group responds by attending to the damsel.

Through the joint creation, the dramatic transformation and the sharing it became clear that the damsel was the real protagonist: the one who knew how to win and lose, who proposed a new beginning in order to survive, who contended in order not to be excluded, who decided what living really meant in order not to die. Thus the protagonic theme is concluded, and returning to the group context allows the emotional interchange and reflections of the personal resonances that occurred within the group.

In the sharing, Renata talks about her mother's preoccupation to avoid her daughter getting hurt. Influenced by this concern of her mother, Renata married a man who was extremely in love with her, as if by doing this she would gain control over her happiness. Her choice of husband was made based on the criterion of safety, which now has been shaken by his betrayal. She neglected her own freedom of choice and her freedom to express her real feelings.

What Daniela shared with the group, was that she was raised to respect the value of the mother and housewife roles. Profession and career have never been seen by her or her family as valuable. She has followed the models of her mother and grandmother, with the consent of her husband and father. She never invested in her career or her professional status; she simply lived a predestined life. Therefore we can conclude that the protagonist of this dramatic act revealed itself through the character of the damsel; in the performance of this character, various roles converged – daughter, betrothed wife, future princess, etc. – confronting the character with conflicts and inquiries, and demanding changes.

Returning to the questions outlined at the beginning of this chapter, now we find ourselves in front of the necessity for a more precise conceptualization of this psychodramatic instrument: the protagonist.

In my definition the protagonist is the element of the dramatic context that arises through the role play of a character; this character questions its own actions and feelings, and is an emotional representative for the relationships established between the members of the group, or between the director and the client, who have a common dramatic aim.

Having conceptualized it in the above manner, now I would like to clearly disconnect the concept of the protagonist from the figure of the individual within the group context, whose complaints or issues justify the proposal for dramatization. When inviting one or more group members (or the client of an individual session) onto the psychodramatic stage, we actually summon authors, who are at the same time the actors of the plot that will develop on this stage. In this process numerous characters are created, and out of these one will stand out through his arguments and feelings and by mobilizing the drama will demand a change. This principal character will become the protagonist.

The figure of the protagonist originates in the Greek tragedy, dating back to the fifth century BC. Before the tragedy, Hellenic myths were represented in religious rituals, as well as epic and lyrical poems, but it was only with the appearance of the tragic man that the social and psychological aspects and conditions of human life started to be expressed. Tragedy is not just simply a literary style; it is a social institution where the city and its citizens are represented, not only to glorify their heroes, but also to question them. The Greek tragedy usually opened with a *chorus* consisting of a group of citizens who, through their comments and chanting, had the role of the narrator, expressing the feelings of the community. Thespis, the first tragic poet (sixth century BC), chose a member of the chorus to incarnate the character of the hero; this chorus member was using masks, not in a ritual way, but to represent the character. This individualized character served to develop the theme, while the chorus continued to chant the feelings. This actor was then accompanied by a second actor, also taken from the chorus, followed by the confrontation of the two characters within the scene. As the scene was further enriched by the entry of other actors, the chorus decreased, changed and eventually lost its original function. Thus, the Greek theatre turns into a public assembly where traditional values are questioned. It is during the enactment that the past becomes present and the distant becomes close. In this tragic perspective the hero always moves on two levels: the level of divine causality and the level of human causality. From Aeschylus to Euripides there was a gradual shift of focus from the divine powers to the powers of man, powers resulting from his feelings and passions. From simply enacting the narrative, the central character of the Greek tragedy moves on to question his own actions. It is this outstanding figure (character) of the Greek tragedy that really interests us. He is the protagonist, the main character of the drama, responsible for the main thread of the action, the main contender (*protagonistes*), the one who will confront the old and the new, the past and the present, the sacred and the profane, the myth and the reality, the one who – accepting the questions and arguments raised by the community – will decipher the enigma of his story.

But who is this protagonist in psychodrama, and how does he emerge? Will the conceptualization of the protagonist be different in a public, group or individual psychodrama or in sociodrama? In order to answer these questions, I will look at the concept of the protagonist through the example of a group supervision session.

The protagonist in psychodrama

A psychodrama trainee, whom I will call A, brought to a supervision session his difficulty of managing a dramatic scene interrupted by his client's crying. From a series of other possible working issues, the group chose A's difficulty to be looked at during supervision. The supervisor suggested the dramatization of what happened in the session directed by A.

On the dramatic stage we have the client (represented by the supervised trainee A) and the therapist (represented by another trainee, whom I will call B).

Scene 1: The therapy room; *present*: client and therapist.

    Client: [addressing the therapist]: I would like to talk to my father about moving out from home, but I know that I will cry and won't manage to carry on.

The therapist suggests the dramatization of this scene.

Scene 2: The living room of the client's house; *present*: father and his daughter (client).

Sitting in front of her father, the daughter says: Father, I will move out from this house, I am looking for my own place; everything has always been only for my sister here... At this point she falls into tears and she cannot say anything else.

The therapist (played by B) does not know how to move on with the scene and so the action is paralysed – just as it happened to therapist A in the real situation.

At this moment of the supervision session, therapist B identifies with therapist A from the real situation, and they both identify with the client. Within the group context the other trainees are wondering what to do. They are all immobilized by the tears of the client, looking at the supervisor and asking for his help. The client's issue was becoming unanimated, the trainee's (A) complaint referred to the interruption of the dramatic scene during the therapy session, while the whole supervision group complained about feeling paralysed. Future, past and present are all there in one single moment. The daughter, the actual client, the dramatic client, the actual therapist, the dramatic therapist, the trainees and the supervisor are all united by a common emotion, by a common aim. The social context (the client's home, A's therapy room) and the group context (the supervision group) are represented in the dramatic context by the *daughter immobilized by tears*. It is this character whom we call protagonist. In the above situation, this protagonist appears in the second scene, when an initially individual problem turns into a collective one. It emerges from the emotional plot that developed in the father–daughter, therapist–client, therapist–client-group and therapist–group–supervisor relationships. Our protagonist is the *man immobilized by his emotions*; it is not the *daughter wanting to leave home*, or *who wants to tell this to her father*, and it is not the *trainee who has difficulties in performing his professional role* either. The aim is no longer to *manage to talk to the father*, to *attend well to a client*, to *learn* or to *teach trainees*. However, these aims will not be annulled, but they will be comprised into a single aim: to be lived and experienced by the protagonist. This protagonist is the main contender, who will confront his own, as well as our immobility. If earlier on we had the text, now – since the plot has been unveiled – we have the subtext, the possibility for renewal.

If – according to the above argument – the protagonist only emerged in the second scene, what did we have until then? Who was this person who appeared – from the group context – in the first scene?

In order to answer this question, let us look at certain situations that may occur in a group. Let us imagine a group member presenting his complaints, feelings, etc.; in response to this, an interaction may develop within the group, leading to a sociometric configuration with this particular group member in its centre, a group member in whom the personal issues of most group members converge. We could say that in this case we have a *group emergent* (or emergent from the group). Other times, there may be an individual who appears to be in crisis, being extremely anxious or depressed, and in need of strong group cohesion. This may evoke the intention of the group to help this suffering group member, *designating* him for dramatic work. There are also other situations when various personal issues are brought to the group, and the psychodramatist will *choose* one of the group members for dramatic work, but without ascertaining the agglutination of the group around one or another issue. In all the above cases however, the *emergent, designated* or *chosen* group member cannot be called protagonist; it is more correct to call him *group representative* (because protagonization is a function of the dramatic context). If we try to find an analogy with the Greek theatre, we could say that what happens in the group context is similar to the epic narrative, its events are similar to the comments of the chorus, and we are at the level of the predestined, of the divine causality. It is in the *as if* of the dramatic context that the ritualistic and protective mask is taken away in order to allow the emergence of a character who is questioning his actions and feelings.

When the therapist-director meets the group representative, or the individual client within the dramatic context, there is an initial phase when the director does most of the action; he asks questions, requests images or scenes and takes the initiative. The attention is focused on him. He is the quack, the saviour, who can solve the presented issue; he is the main contender, the dramatic intention being most strongly represented by him. Therefore we can say that the initial protagonization is that of the director; it is through the warm-up and the initial scenes the director will allow the protagonic activity to shift to the characters emerging from the dramatization. We often work with scenes that have a low emotional intensity and little spontaneity (for example, the investigation of the social atom, the interview, the marking of something), which demand constant intervention from the director. Other scenes, a keyword, or an evoked feeling may mobilize the emotional forces inside the client, the therapist and the group, propitiating the director to identify the protagonist. This leads to a dramatic flow, making the director's figure less visible for the group and the client; now the therapist becomes incorporated in the action, playing together with the protagonist.

Originating in the co-conscious and co-unconscious states and the common dramatic aim (representing emotionally the relationships established between the participants of the session), here is the one who questions, argues, deciphers, changes, and fights in the common drama. This is the *real protagonist*; while all the elements preceding it could be called *pre-protagonists* or *intermediary protagonists*.

In processual therapies there are sessions that have a descriptive, comprehensive or warm-up character, the scenes consisting of these pre-protagonic elements. Other times we may have group themes, with issues around the inter-relations of the participants or issues of an inter-group kind; in such cases we say that the client is the group, and we have the possibility of working with or without a protagonist.

I mentioned earlier on that what happens in the group context is similar to the epic narrative; however, there are sessions that develop on a verbal level and after defining the *emergent*, the rest of the group will either take the position of the spectator or that of an interlocutor. In these cases, if we have a narrative made up of facts, the presentation of feelings or questioning of the plot, and all this leads to the emotional involvement of the participants (with the person who narrates), we could say that even in the absence of classical dramatization, the group context becomes dramatic. The dramatic structure is present: on the one hand we have the narrator, who will turn himself into a character, and on the other hand we have the group, at times silently watching and witnessing what is happening, other times asking questions, making statements, expressing feelings (similar to the Greek chorus). The epic turns into *tragedy*.

I would also like to stress the importance of the therapist's spectator-participant function within group sessions and especially in individual sessions. Through his affective attachment (at times identification), the therapist intrigues himself with the plot, he listens because he wants to know more, he asks to get involved, he becomes an accomplice in order for the story to become a *drama*. This inter-subjectivity will support the emotional climate, demanding a common aim; it will be the guide for the potagonic movement. This will then move on to a succession of characters, roles, relationships, feelings.

The protagonic movement (theme) is already present in the group context; however, it is in the dramatic context where the *protagonist* will emerge. The scene is the protagonist's *locus nascendi*, being interrelational is its *matrix*, and it is through this that author, actor and character all become one single element. Considering that the protagonist is one of the main pillars of psychodrama, we can conclude that it is through its definition that theatre becomes therapeutic, that it turns into creative revolution.

Note

1 Originally published under the title 'O protagonista e o tema protagônico'. In W.C. Almeida (1999) *Grupos – A Proposta do Psicodrama [Groups – Proposal for Psychodrama]*. São Paulo: Ágora, pp.89–100.

9

The theatre of spontaneity and psychodrama psychotherapy[1]

Moysés Aguiar

In order to discuss this topic, I would like to propose the use of the following two theoretical tools: the concept of the *dramatic project* and the concept of *focus-and-shade*.

The concept of *dramatic project* allows us a theoretical approximation between the sociometric instruments and the theatrical aspect of psychodrama. The dramatic project is an application and expansion of the 'criterion' concept of the sociometric test within the social, group and psychodramatic contexts. It is based on the hypothesis that the forces of attraction and repulsion (forming a field of relationships) are established in the function of a multitude of interdependent criteria, which collectively catalyse the group.

This catalysing effect involves not only a teleological variable (or in other words, the global objectives of the group), but also a set of partial goals of different levels, as well as an arsenal of established instruments that are applied by the group in order to make their goals feasible. Material means, as well as resources of an ethical, aesthetic, behavioural and relational order are all included within this set of instruments. The totality of these components constitutes the dramatic project of the group.

The dramatic project as a reference presides the distribution of roles among the various group members, creating the conditions for the individual actions to jointly lead to the desired objectives. It defines expectations regarding the behaviour and the ways in which tools such as norms, values, technology, creativity, leadership, power, etc. are going to be used.

Since the dramatic project is an essentially collective phenomenon (the building of a collective product), casual individual 'dramatic projects' (attributed to a specific group member), do not fit into this perspective of the dramatic project. Thus, when we try to understand a phenomenon through the prism of socionomy, it is important to take into consideration the dramatic project of the examined entity; this will allow the evaluation of those aspects of the tele-relationships that will mark the role-performance.

It is also important not to fragment the object of our examination, neither to look at its decomposed parts in isolation from their global, direct and dynamic reality. For this reason it is appropriate to look at the concepts of *focus* and *shade*, when working with the idea of the dramatic project. The term 'focus' was introduced by Moreno (1946) in connection with the concept of psychosomatic roles. According to him, within this role category, one of the partners (the infant) is unable to fully apprehend the relational other (or 'Thou') in its totality; he will perceive only those fragments of the other, which the infant's neurological maturity allows. It is this partial perception that Moreno called focus.

This Morenian categorization is actually a bit unfortunate, because – due to its imprecise formulation – it allowed taking into consideration only one part of the relationship (the child) instead of looking at the relationship as a whole. As a consequence, the multi-polarity of the role concept (which is at least dual) also became jeopardized, once the assumption was taken that a role could be understood considering only the perspective of one of the people involved. This is a theoretical mistake.

Focus is also often used in theatre as one of the main tools of scenic communication. Let us imagine a stage with various actors on it, each one of them performing their character. Simultaneous micro-scenes unfold on this stage. A strong light beam can be projected onto one of these scenes, directing the spectator's attention towards it, leaving all the other scenes in dim light. This dim light can also be applied when the actors are in a waiting posture within the scenic space, or it can be used to provide continuity for the presentation, while the change of costumes or scenery takes place. This strategy is a technical alternative: when not being involved in the action, instead of leaving the stage (moving to the sides), the actors may remain there, in the shade, or 'out of focus'.

The implicit meta-message within this scenery is that while certain things happen in a certain place, at the same time others are happening in another space and these latter are also part of the plot. Since it is impossible to look at everything at the same time, we need to choose where to direct (focus) the attention. This technique has also been used by painters such as Rembrandt and his school.

This interaction between focus and shade can be seen as a form of editing reality, which allows us to overcome the risk of fragmentation. Within this interaction the part clearly belongs to the whole; we are reminded that although the attention is directed to a specific aspect, there are also other aspects that are part of the examined fact, without being dissociated from it.

Through the above considerations I intended to establish the pretext of this – still preliminary – reflection regarding the diverse forms of action within the professional space of psychodrama. In order to map out this diversity, I will first look at the various 'dramatic projects' established within the different forms of psychodrama practise, trying to identify what is in the 'focus' of each one of these projects. A psychodrama director needs to establish and/or direct himself towards a specific focus within his work. He aims to enlighten a specific facet of the situation representing the object of the psychodramatic work. This doesn't mean that he will deny the existence of other aspects; he will only leave these in the shade (or even to the side), while prioritizing the chosen facets.

This option of the director determines his choice of the technical resources that he will use within the work. Consequently, it also defines the theoretical requirements of the psychodramatic work, not only stimulating the director's cogitation, but also his motivation for the research of bibliography, and possible complementary skills.

When striving for a greater interchange between the different versions of psychodrama initially there will probably be more to exchange between those areas which have the same focus, compared to those that prioritize different focuses. The reason for this is that approaches with the same focus share their fundamental assumptions; while in the case of approaches with divergent focuses, it is exactly these basic assumptions that are argued.

Diagnostic psychodrama: focus on pathology

The intention within this approach is to take the complaint of the client and to redescribe it in terms of previously established categories; these categories are both the instruments and the fruits of the investigations. Such categories will shape the tools through which knowledge is obtained (*dia* = through; *gnosis* = knowledge), and propitiate a guideline for the treatment. The diagnosis can focus on the individual, the group or the relationships. When focusing on the individual, at least two separate models can be adopted: the psychiatric and the psychological model.

The psychiatric model corresponds to the traditional medical perspective that works with nosological categories, trying to include the patient into one of them and then to establish a therapeutic conduct and prognosis. In this case, psychodramatic resources replace the conventional form of anamnesis and clinical observation, and provide a richer and more dynamic knowledge compared to the purely verbal interview.

The psychological model focuses on the psychological characteristics of the client, aiming to provide a description as detailed and precise as possible of the personality traces as well as the psychodynamics of the individual. Needless to say, personality and psychodynamics can be evaluated according to different theoretical references. In a psychodramatic diagnosis, the psychodramatist can resort to any of these available theoretical reference points, or he can even try to apply a socionomic perspective. This effort to apply a socionomic point of reference will also imply an attempt to find an alternative psychiatric model, a kind of psychodramatic psychopathology.

When shifting the focus from the individual to the group, it is possible to apply the same basic diagnostic format, by looking at the group as an individuality in itself that transcends the members of which it consists. However, categorical models cannot always be transposed from one universe to another in the same format as they were originally conceived. Thus, the diagnostic categories used for the definition of individual pathologies, can only be used for the description of groups if appropriately 'recycled'. Alternatively, new categories need to be created that are appropriate to the new scope of investigation (the group); in this case the group diagnosis will have its own language and its specific procedures.

In order to succeed, diagnosis will depend on this mapping which, if not established previously, should be done as the therapeutic process advances. The better the precision and validity of diagnosis, the bigger the chances for helping the patient.

This diagnostic perspective ignores some of the basic assumptions of existential philosophy, which are usually attributed to psychodrama. This is due to the fact that, within the diagnostic approach, the nosological instances are considered to be the 'essence': the complaint of a specific patient represents a particular case of a general occurrence. 'Existence' – while it is unique to the client – remains in the shade; the focus is directed onto the non-unique, onto the category.

In our practise, the psychodramatic technique of 'interviewing a character' has a diagnostic focus; originally however, it had the function of warming-up the protagonist and/or bringing out the subtext of the text. Within its diagnostic application, the interview is carried out by the director while the protagonist is in the dramatic context; however, the interview happens without actual dramatization. The questions represent a form of interviewing which is different from what would be used in a usual verbal anamnesis: we don't only question the character representing the client, but also his/her partners (counter-roles) – this creates the conditions for obtaining clearer information regarding the problem which we are investigating.

A possible difficulty that may occur in this kind of interview is that – under the weight of the obtained information, without arriving to formulate a diagnosis, and under the tacit obligation to 'pay back' this information earned with hard work – the director may end up with a very few options for how to proceed with the enactment. Even if he manages to draw a conclusion (diagnosis), the director will need to confront another dilemma, since merely telling the diagnosis to the client will not solve the problem.

According to these operational models, once the diagnosis is defined, we should move on to the therapy: once the illness is defined, we have to prescribe the medicine. And that suggests to the psychodramatist that – in order to proceed with his work – he should resort to another 'focus'.

Gestalt psychodrama: focus on the perception

Gestalt therapy, developed by Fritz Perls' school, introduced numerous aspects that don't just exclusively belong to the gestalt approach. The gestalt theory distinguished itself by discovering the general laws of perception. Its epistemological postulates are in contraposition to those of the atomism (from the end of the nineteenth century, these latter were very influential for the development of scientific psychological research).

The thesis of gestalt theory is that the mind functions through configurations: stimuli are organized by the person who perceives them in such a manner that they 'acquire' a form. Certain forms impose themselves onto the person, because within the field of the object the stimuli are already arranged in a sufficiently structured manner. In other cases, when on the 'objective' level (the field of the object) the stimuli are arranged in a more ambiguous and less structured manner, the perceptive organizations will reflect much stronger the 'subjective' structures of the person.

The way an individual moves in the world is marked by the form the world is perceived by him. This model could also be applied to other areas of the psyche, such as the memory, intelligence, learning, thinking, self-image, etc. Any behavioural change is conditioned by a reconfiguration which the person should carry out concerning himself, others, the world and relationships. Such modifications of perception would have immediate effects on all other mental processes, including feelings. As part of this general reorganization and as a result of the change in the way the individual 'sees' things, the behaviour will also change.

By providing their clients with the possibility to focus on certain aspects of life that are in the 'background' (or 'shade') and so change them into 'form', gestalt therapy attempts to revolutionize the relationships of the individual. The therapeutic work proceeds with the revision of rigid perceptive structures in such a way that new information is incorporated into these structures and new configurations are built.

As perception essentially has a subjective component (it is impossible for the 'exterior' environment to exclusively determine the structure of what an individual perceives), any change within the person will necessarily determine a new gestalt for the previous perceptions about the world.

This effect is circular: a change in the perception leads to a change in the individual, which in turn changes the perception, and so on. This perspective can also be adopted in psychodrama: the psychodrama session enfolds, having as its objective to guide the participants towards a reconfiguration of their perception regarding their life and their problems.

When the dramatization in itself is not sufficient to achieve this result, psychodramatists often transform the sharing into a phase of comments, discussion and reflection. The therapist 'points out' certain aspects of the client's behaviour that became evident in the previous phases of the session, thus complementing the client's experience from the stage, by showing him a different, new and reorganized structure, which is sufficiently strong to unchain a re-creation of his perception.

It is usual to pair up this approach with diagnostic psychodrama; the client will review both the diagnostic conclusions and observations made by the therapist. It is expected that once his perception of the problem has been changed, the client's reactions to conflicts will also change.

One of the most frequent hindrances to the efficiency of this method is when the therapist manages to obtain an understanding of the phenomenon, but without ensuring that the gestalt formulated by him is also understood by the client. Or, what is even more intriguing, is when the client manages to see what is demonstrated to him, but without this new understanding having any immediate visible influence on his behaviour.

Reparatory psychodrama: focus on the history

According to the more popular psychotherapeutic currents, the problems that individuals need to confront originate in their personal history, in facts that happened a long time ago. These approaches emphasize the more primitive episodes: the earlier an experience, the greater its influence on later development. As a consequence, these approaches attempt to find out what happened in the early stages of life which would justify the blunders of the present. This approach is so strongly rooted in our culture that many people when asked what brought them to therapy, do not refer to their present everyday conflicts and difficulties, but complain about a 'problematic childhood', 'problems within their primary family', 'childhood traumas', etc.

In its early stages of development psychodrama wasn't so concerned with these historical aspects; this perspective was incorporated into psychodrama during its later development. Nowadays it has become so important that many psychodramatists mistake it for the actual idea of psychodrama.

Williams (1989) pointed it out that Moreno himself preferred a 'horizontal' approach; it was Zerka's great interest for psychotic patients that contributed to the development of a 'vertical' approach. By *verticalization* we mean a historical-etiological research; what gives an investigation a vertical character, is the ability to transcend the superficiality, to transcend the more apparent.

Moreno introduced the concept of 'second time', considered by Fanchette (1986) to be the basic structure of the psychodramatic method. According to Fanchette, the 'repetition' of a traumatic event allows the individual to overcome and master it; this process is similar to the shamanic dances of primitive man that were used to exorcise his fears and to dominate the powers of nature, with which he was confronted.

This is one of the modalities of reparatory action in psychodrama: to identify crucial past events or incidents and represent them on the stage. Re-experiencing the feelings that are associated to this event will allow a fading of its strength and a decrease of its relative importance in the present life.

Another alternative is to reproduce the event within the dramatic context, looking for a different outcome. When a new ending can be experimented with, the fragility of the client – revealed by his failure to satisfactorily solve an adverse past situation – will give way to the power of the present. This effect can be achieved through a simple catharsis. The 'purification' achieved through this process liberates the client, who acquires the conditions for performing his life without the weight of this useless burden.

There is also another possibility for finding a new solution to the old conflict; a solution that is different from the one that the client presented. At a certain point of the story we start to re-tell it, leading it towards a new ending, which is happier that the previous one.

We need to remember that the traumatic event had happened in another context: technically speaking, in the social context. As such, by definition this event is situated in the realm of 'real'(ity) in the sense that Moreno attributed to this term. The reproduction of the event however, is within the dramatic context, in the 'as if', within the realm of the imaginary.

Therefore, the enactment of this event will necessarily involve re-creation. As a consequence, one may question whether what happened in the past is exactly and correctly told by the client, as well as whether the scene presented on the stage faithfully reproduces the fact which it intends to represent. We may also question whether this intention is feasible.

However, what is really important within the dramatic context is that the essential outlines of the past event are reproduced in such a way that this will generate the same emotions as the ones originally evoked by the event itself. This is sufficient in order to obtain the effect of repetition–reformulation.

When investigating this crucial scene, there is a choice of using two different 'focuses'. One of them searches for that initial event which can be considered the first link within the causal chain. In this case, we talk about regressive psychodrama, which intends to recede in time and through a sequence of scenes to arrive at a nodal scene. After having reached this objective, it returns to the current conflict, re-examining the problem under a new light directed on reparation.

The second possible focus discards the idea of causality and considers the scene as merely paradigmatic, and not as 'determinant' of the present difficulties. These difficulties are seen as the visible manifestations of a complex of historical forces, forming an integrated and lasting system. The 'traumatic' event is simply a symbol/synthesis of the way these forces act and are structured. Therefore, this event is not necessarily the oldest at which we can arrive.

Technically speaking, it may have the same value as a totally and assumedly imaginary or fictitious scene, because the structure of relationships can also become apparent under such circumstances. In the case of both focuses, the psychodramatic experience is considered as a possibility to repair something that has gone awry, and which currently manifests itself in difficulties, causing pain and suffering.

In reparatory psychodrama the psycho- or socio-pathological aspect is in the scene at all times, although a previous diagnosis is not always considered essential. The symptoms can be considered as a guide that will lead to the real problem (a problem that is situated beyond the symptoms), these symptoms being always referred to the history, to a broader temporal process.

Pragmatic psychodrama: focus on the there-outside

In contrast with reparatory psychodrama, which considers the present difficulty to be a particular manifestation of a background problem, pragmatic psychodrama prefers to look at the client's complaint as a problem that needs to be solved. This approach does not distinguish between the symptom and the illness; the latter is considered to be the symptom itself. It does not talk about pathology, but considers the presented complaints to be a situation of impasse or a lack of ability.

Therefore, the director suggests the problematic situation to be brought into the dramatic context, in the most direct and 'objective' way possible. Through the use of various resources this approach tries to make an adequate equation of the problem, investigating its antecedents, amplitude and its implications. The climax of this kind of work is the formulation of various hypotheses regarding possible solutions. The intention is to achieve a resolution within the dramatic context that is satisfactory enough in order to be carried forward and applied within the social context.

However, psychodrama also has other applications within this pragmatic focus. There are situations for example, where the problem as well as its practical solution is already clearly defined, and so what is necessary is to prepare the client for the satisfactory application of this solution. In this case we talk about spontaneity training that is carried out through role-playing. The applied procedures are already more or less defined; what is required from the client is not only to recognize the expectations, but also a certain degree of ease and freedom in order to handle the matter.

Feelings that may obstruct a good performance are only dealt with on a more superficial level, the intention being to leave the path unobstructed, while there is no attempt made for a deeper and more profound understanding of the meaning of these feelings. What is important is to encourage spontaneity.

Play is a healthy exercise for the fantasy, which enriches the repertoire of alternative responses; one of theses responses may prove to be useful. It also plays an encouraging part in the effective application of some solutions, of which the client already has got a glimpse, but is unable to apply them.

Due to its similarities to the behavioural approach, pragmatic psychodrama gives gooseflesh to certain professionals and has lead to numerous criticisms. It is often considered a superficial approach, without any perspective for real change. The counter-argument is that any alteration within the sequence of facts may result in an inflection or change of the causal chain and it may reflect in the phenomena that are interconnected with the causal chain. Furthermore, when successfully applied, pragmatic psychodrama liberates spontaneity and creativity.

Spontaneous theatre: focus on the creation

In the scenes that are put under this spotlight the main intention is to propitiate the opportunity to create a dramatic representation. In creative psychodrama the role of the director consists in the facilitation, stimulation and implementation of creation. He facilitates the embryonic ideas brought to the session being made into scenes, and as these are enacted, he will encourage the search for new ideas in order to allow the gradual building up of the plot. The solution or closure of the narrative is not considered as a guideline for the future that should be adopted in the social context; it only serves the dramatic context.

In its form, spontaneous theatre is similar to entertainment-theatre (or art-theatre), searching for resources of development and improvement. At a superficial glance it may seem similar to infantile games, without any major implications, responsibility or seriousness. In spite of this, however, spontaneous theatre constitutes a respectable and widely applied form of therapy and learning.

While this working modality may privilege the protagonist as the focus of dramatic production, it will not concern itself with his psyche as such. The protagonist's feelings, fantasies, reactions, etc. represent the raw material for the creation of the plot, however, they do not consist of the object of analysis, trial, judgement or interpretation. The therapeutic-pedagogic effect consists in the mere participation in a collective creation process, associated with the effort of investigating reality. It is the process what matters, not the product.

The underlying conflict – the condition for the construction of a dramatic text – is defined as the scene builds up, while the effort to construct a plot enables an investigation of reality as well as the investigation of its real contradictions. The working hypothesis is: even though the apparent content of the dramatic account may seem imaginary, through this story we can identify those relational structures that reside in the life of the participants, and therefore, in the life of the protagonist itself. Furthermore, when enacting the maps of their realities, through the spontaneous creation of scenes, people can question them. The great gain is not the conscience of the conflict in itself, but the opportunity to do something about it in a creative manner.

Experimenting with different attitudes and believing in their capacity to create and test how joyful creation can be, is a transforming experience for all the participants, regardless of the modality of scenic representation we use: lyrical, epical or comical.

Some authors made references to the ancient Greek tragedy, whose literary structure contains a dialectic play as an important element of linking up the narrative. With this, they warn against certain risks such as chaotic and unstructured representations where the characters enter and exit the scene without any engagement in the collective production, as if it was a spontaneous act.

As the objective of this chapter is to explore this particular focus characteristic to the spontaneous theatre, in the following I will look in more detail at some of its most important aspects.

Psychodrama and the theatre of spontaneity

It is inevitable for us psychodramatists to discuss the relationship between psychodrama and theatre. There are various approaches to this relationship: at one extreme we have the premise that psychodrama and theatre have nothing in common, while on the other there is a tendency to have theatre as the main emphasis. The former of these represent an attitude of 'I don't know and I don't care about it', while the latter an attitude of 'I don't know about it, but I like it'. Spontaneous theatre was born out of an aesthetic anxiety, as a consequence of questioning the classical theatre, and a proposal of a new alternative.

The theatre of spontaneity is at the root of psychodrama. As Moreno started to recognize and discover its therapeutic effects, he gradually transformed the original theatre of spontaneity into 'classical' psychodrama.

Nevertheless, the theatre of spontaneity continues to be the basic technique for what we include under the umbrella of psychodrama. In this respect, spontaneous theatre is not just simply a particular modality or technique within the wide spectrum of possibilities in the psychodrama practise, as people often assume.

Psychodrama can be understood as the theatre of spontaneity providing growth to the individual members within a group. It differs from sociodrama, which also uses the spontaneous theatre, but its subject is a preexistent, 'natural' group and its objective is the growth of the group as a whole.

Let us now see some of the characteristics of the spontaneous theatre.

The dramatic action

Since the theatre of spontaneity is a form of dramatic art, it cannot exist without action. However, it isn't just concerned with any action – and this is where psychodrama differs from other action techniques.

By definition, theatre presupposes two fundamental components: the stage and the audience. On the stage stories are acted out by actors, and these stories are watched and seen by the spectators. There are numerous possibilities to create links between these two elements, but we can never give up one for the other, because if this happened, theatre would cease being theatre.

What defines the specificity of the spontaneous theatre is improvisation. In its closest form to classical psychodrama, it does not have a pre-written text: the *script* is co-created by the actors and spectators as it is being enacted. There are however, also other possibilities, such as working with already written texts, interpreting and enacting them (as for example, in dramatherapy, or in Brecht's 'Learning Play'); or when the presentation is done only by professional actors (for example, playback theatre).

Under ideal circumstances, the enactment is characterized by the protagonist's state of being-out-of-himself, a rupture with rationality and control, an adventure into the unknown, into the irrational. Participants of dramatizations often report about this experience of transient 'madness', about their sense of loss for the content, a loss of factual memory regarding what happened during the scene.

Theatre of spontaneity requires full involvement from all group members, with a shared responsibility for what is going to happen. This involvement usually results in powerful experiences, with all participants feeling touched and experiencing some sort of potentially transforming impact. When achieving this degree of involvement, psychodrama becomes more active, displaying an elevated level of emotional and aesthetic involvement.

It is not only the protagonist, who is in the focus of the group, but also those participants who enter the stage in order to perform other roles; and even those who remain in the audience. Thus, the therapeutic potential of the action is maximized.

Co-creation

In the theatre of spontaneity the act is the participation; act may or may not involve speech, but it is certainly more than just words. However, this is not a solitary act; through over-exposure or unilateral denudation and de-contextualization, a solitary act would have the risk of turning into exhibitionism or moral suicide. The act is a collective process of constructing an art product, an improvised theatrical performance.

This experience provides the discovery of ways for living together; each moment of this experience demands a flexible, inventive and engaged participation in the group process, with a balanced way of addressing both collective and individual needs, an equilibrium based on spontaneity and creativity. The perspective and the approach characteristic of the spontaneous theatre favours the participation of everybody in the creative process, giving a great opportunity for inter-personal relationships to develop and to be better understood.

Content

The content is always and necessarily a topic that is connected to the personal life of each participant as an individual, interconnected with certain relevant aspects of community life. It doesn't matter if it is wrapped in the 'real facts from the life of the protagonist', 'a collective quotidian anecdote' or an 'assumingly fantasy story'. An issue brought into a session by an individual, may be seen both as something that belongs only to him/her (molecular view), or as an expression of a transpersonal whole that reaches beyond the life of the individual (molar view). The story narrated on the stage is always the fruit of the imaginary, even if it claims or aspires to faithfully reproduce real-life events. At the same time, even if in the moment it is understood as if its starting point is the 'total imaginary', this story is inspired by 'real' life.

Moreno intended to cure through the repetition of traumatic events within the scenic space; however, I believe that nothing repeats itself: every dramatization is a creation of a new story, even if it claims to reproduce the old. Far from being a limitation, Moreno's approach is actually liberating, because it opens up a much wider horizon: everything that is created is able to put people in touch with deeper and more profound aspects of the reality of their life.

Since the perspective is always analogical, it is possible to obtain an image of the system represented through the dramatization; to obtain a picture of some of the forces that are involved, that interact and to a certain extent explain those facets of life that were brought into the focus in that moment of the dramatization.

Art as a reference point

Spontaneous theatre is a form of art, a process that addresses reality, aiming to reach a certain kind of understanding or knowledge. Art however, aims to obtain a different kind of knowledge than the scientific methods.

In contrast with the scientific approaches, the fundamental condition or criteria of art is to prioritize the intuitive, the original expression and the aesthetic as ways to enable the individual to experience, without necessarily using reason. This experientially gained knowledge can have the same or an even stronger transforming effect than rationally obtained knowledge. However, the therapeutic effect of art is only secondary, because the main objective of art is art itself.

So, what does it mean to adopt art as a reference point for the therapeutic practise? First of all, it means that creativity should have a privileged space within the therapeutic situation. The therapist should be daring and sensitive to the uniqueness of each moment; he/she should be able to transform this sensitivity into proposals for action, thus creating a climate that is strongly characterized by creativity. At the same time, the client should be encouraged to abandon his/her repetitive ways of action and thinking and to become more and more daring. Art cannot exist without a daring and bold attitude and without 'self-surprises'. This is also true for therapy.

In the theatre of spontaneity, this creativity is implemented through techniques that are characteristic of this artistic modality. The range of these techniques incorporates resources that are in full evolution and transformation.

The function of spontaneous theatre is to structure a situation in such way, that it doesn't leave room for routine, because routine can endanger the session.

The director is required to use his/her sensitivity in order to perceive what every moment demands, and to respond to these demands with maximum invention. The approach of the spontaneous theatre opens the doors of aesthetics in psychotherapy. If this criterion is incorporated in the practise of psychodrama, it will influence the therapist's ability to go 'straight to the point' and to propitiate an intense emotional experience. In order to achieve an aesthetic effect every small detail is important: in order to develop an art-psychodrama (or psychodrama-art) we need to invest a lot in its technical aspects, but taking good care not to create a gap between the theory and practise.

A rational complement

Another question is whether it is sufficient to propose an artistic activity without complementing it with a kind of cognitive dessert following this action-based, emotional meal.

This is a question frequently raised by professionals who use Piagetian elements in their work, and based on their research regarding intellectual development are convinced that the learning process cannot be complete without reaching reason. From a strictly artistic point of view, such a rational formulation becomes unnecessary; any attempt to translate these discoveries into another form of communication, would bring about an impoverishment. It would be similar to try and explain a joke: trying to intellectually understand a joke, would strip its humour from it. The same is true for dance, music, painting, sculpture, cinema, theatre and literature that uses words in its own original way.

From this artistic perspective we will need to reconsider the traditional necessity of many therapists to make interpretations. This also leaves open the question regarding the phase of sharing, often considered both by the participants and the professionals as a phase for comments, as a moment of analysis, of punctuation, of devolution and of practical suggestions.

Conclusions

Now I would like to return to the question of the different foci within psychodramatic work. As professionals, we move with more or less flexibility between these alternatives, favouring one or another focus in different moments of our work. All these foci represent an infinite number of conceptual and technical problems that would need to be resolved in order to achieve their compatibility with the so-called basic psychodrama, as well as to improve their effectiveness and efficiency. Being stuck on only one of these foci is in contradiction with the very principle of spontaneity–creativity. Also, if in its relationship with the shade, we let the focus turn into exclusive reality, or if we let it become an organically dissociated fragment, it will lose its essence.

When analysing the various foci from the perspective of their scientific productivity, methodological consistence, epistemic coherence or any other parameter that can be applied to scientific processes, we should respect the uniqueness of them all, without trying to homogenize them. Don't forget that psychodrama can also be looked at from a non-scientific, but artistic perspective, in which case its quality will be evaluated based on aesthetic values.

Note

1   Original title: 'O teatro espontâneo e a psicoterapia psicodramática'. Previously unpublished paper.

Part 3

Innovative techniques in Brazilian psychodrama

This final section of the book focuses on the innovative techniques developed and introduced by Brazilian psychodramatists.

Luis Altenfelder presents his psychodramatic work with drawings. He called this technique 'psychogram', that is, the representation of the psyche through graphic images. His chapter gives a description of the technique and presents its use through clinical examples, also giving indications for its application.

Maria Amalia Faller Vitale focuses on the psychodramatic potential of the 'genogram', a tool recognized and widely used by family and couple therapists. The author introduces 'genodrama', the dramatization of the genogram, and discusses the therapeutic process with couples from a sociodramatic perspective.

In the chapter entitled 'Dramatic multiplication', Pedro Mascarenhas gives account of the development, description and application of the dramatic multiplication technique. The author also draws parallels between Moreno's clinical case known as 'the psychodrama of Adolf Hitler' and dramatic multiplication, emphasizing the importance of spontaneous and creative states, the co-unconscious and the aesthetic pleasure of the collective creation.

Rosa Cukier and Sonia Marmelsztejn present their experiences of working psychodramatically with borderline clients. They give a detailed description of the diagnostic characteristics, aetiology and psychodynamics of this personality disorder, explaining why working with this client group can be challenging and suggesting a possible psychodramatic approach for their therapy.

In the next chapter, focusing on sociometry, Antonio Ferrara presents two modalities for the evaluation of the perceptive test and its indices (perception index, emission index, tele index, and the index of group tele). He introduces the graphic representations proposed by Dalmiro Bustos, as well as an alternative modality of tabular representation, allowing an easier calculation and evaluation of these indexes.

Finally, Ronaldo Pamplona da Costa presents his research on Moreno's proposal for the use of therapeutic motion pictures and television. The author describes his own experiences with the making and use of therapeutic films and their presentations on closed circuit as well as open television. He demonstrates that, what was once considered a Morenian utopia may well turn into reality at the beginning of the new millennium.

10

Psychogram
The use of drawings in psychodrama psychotherapy[1]

Luis Altenfelder

The soul never thinks without an image (Aristotle, *De Anima*)

The objective of this chapter is to present the use of drawings combined with other psychodramatic resources used in psychotherapy sessions.

The idea first came to me when I read about psychodrama sessions in which the authors had used drawings for describing scenes. Word, posture, movement and scenery completed each other, forming a meaningful whole and making the story more alive and comprehensible. I started to think about the possibility of using drawings in my own work in order to facilitate my clients' descriptions of images and scenes of their internal world, as if it were an actual dramatization.

Certain people, mainly those to whom control over their environment is important in order to feel secure, show difficulties when asked to dramatize. Dramatization may trigger in them a fear of losing control and the emergence of anxiety, which will block spontaneity. Dramatizations done in such cases are often poor and interrupted by verbal story telling. I started to ask clients who were showing these characteristics to draw. As a result, their story became more alive and powerful, and at times the scenes that were drawn were even re-experienced. Through the means of the drawings, the clients' fear diminished and they became more relaxed; I also noticed that drawings worked as a warm-up process, as a device initiating spontaneous processes, thus overcoming resistance.

I also used drawings with clients unable to participate in dramatizations due to their physical limitations such as paraplegia, arthritis, a heart deficiency, risk of abortion, etc. This technique also worked well when working in a small consultation room, where due to the lack of physical space, a classic dramatization would have been impossible.

I have been working with this technique for nearly five years. I coined it 'psychogram', or in other words, the representation of the psyche through graphic images. According to the Novo Dicionário Aurelio (Buarque de Holanda 1975), the word 'psychogram' means: the description or analysis of the personality. Jaspers (1979) also uses this expression as a record of all biographical findings, presented in an orderly diagram. However, my use of the term 'psychogram' does not coincide with either of the above definitions; but since I couldn't find a more adequate label for this technique, I decided to keep it.

Description of the technique

Psychogram is a 'dramatization' done with drawings. The materials we use in this technique are sheets of paper and pencils or pens. There is no need for the standardization of the material.

Psychodramatic techniques such as soliloquy and role reversal can be applied in a similar manner to classic dramatization. In soliloquy, the protagonist focuses on himself and talks about himself; it is used in order to reproduce hidden feelings and thoughts related to a certain situation, and it has its foundation in the phase of the recognition of the I. In the technique of role reversal, the protagonist takes on the role of the other (and the other the role of the protagonist); this technique is connected to the developmental phase when the child reverses roles with the 'other' of the relationship. Since, when using psychogram there is no 'other' with whom to do an actual role reversal, I prefer to call this technique (following the proposal of Navarro and his colleagues) 'taking the role of the other' (Navarro *et al.* 1978).

The double technique is applied when the protagonist does not manage to bring to the surface (express) some of his feelings and emotions; for its use we need the presence of an auxiliary ego, and for this reason its application may be more impaired when working with the psychogram. The double technique is related to the stage of all identity, the first developmental phase of the child within the matrix of identity (Fonseca 1980).

The mirror technique consists in making the protagonist see himself from a distance, as if watching himself in a mirror; it is based in the developmental phase of the recognition of the I. In a traditional dramatization, this technique is applied when the protagonist does not manage to see or perceive himself. So it requires an auxiliary ego, who will act as the protagonist. The psychogram in itself is close to being a permanent mirror.

Other psychodrama techniques, such as concretization, symbolization, interview, interpretation from inside a role and the dream technique (onirodrama) can also be applied within the psychogram (Bustos 1974; Moreno 1974; Wolff 1981).

In one-to-one therapy situations, the use of the psychogram can at times be more advantageous than classic dramatization. The internal images, expressed through drawings, are genuine creations of the patient. When working with these drawings we don't have the limitation of the one-to-one psychodrama psychotherapy, where (in the absence of an auxiliary ego) the different roles need to be marked or represented by objects that can be found in the therapy room (Campedelli 1978).

My intention is to present the psychogram as an instrument of psychotherapeutic psychodrama. As an illustration, in the following I will describe a few sessions where I used this technique.

Case example: Martha

Martha (30 years old) came for therapy with phobic symptoms, which had become so limiting that she couldn't leave the house anymore unless accompanied by someone. She seemed to be very tense, anxious and shy, with her spontaneity strongly impaired.

She had already been in therapy for around a month, and was usually very tense during sessions. In the therapy room she usually chose to sit on a chair which was behind a table. Her speech was reduced to the description of her symptoms: tremors, tachycardia, diaphoresis, feelings of pre-cordial pressure and other physical signs of anxiety. Fear became a central and dominating issue in her life. She responded with fear to my proposals for dramatization and so these suggestions were refused by her saying: 'I am afraid to lose control'.

In the session that I describe, Martha was as tense and shaky as usual and she only talked about her symptoms. We were both sat at the table, facing each other, and I asked Martha to take a pencil and a piece of paper and draw herself. First she was a bit perplexed and said that she couldn't draw, but eventually drew an outline (Figure 10.1). Here I used the technique of symbolization as a construction of a static image (Bustos 1974). Following this, I asked her to draw how she was feeling at the moment (Figure 10.2). While she was drawing, I attempted to describe the drawing: it was a sense of tremor and dizziness, a bad feeling, a fear that did not leave her in peace.

Figure 10.1 Martha's drawing of herself

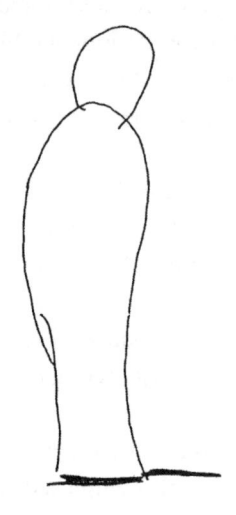

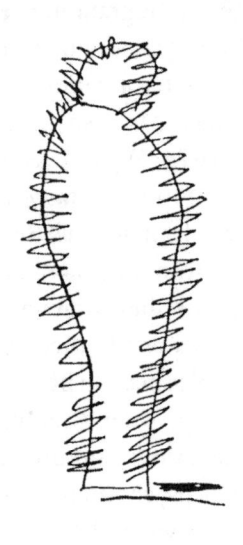

Figure 10.2 Martha's representation of herself; the bold line at the outlines of her body is the concretization of her feelings

Here, I proceeded in a way similar to the technique of concretization. The visualization of the symptom through the drawing allowed us to focus our attention on that aspect in which the conflict probably manifested itself (externalized), this being followed by the investigation of its roots. According to Fonseca (1980), through the concretization of an internal image, its therapeutic handling becomes easier.

I asked Martha to talk as if she was the tremor (to take on the role of the tremor). In order to facilitate the conversation, I encouraged her to continue drawing the symptom and to keep on drawing during the conversation:

Therapist: What are you doing to Martha?

Martha: [in the role of her tremor]: I am making her feel bad.

Therapist: Why?

Tremor: To show that she is afraid.

Therapist: Afraid of what?

Tremor: Of being alone.

At this point Martha had got out of role and interrupted the conversation. She told me that she always had this fear. She remembered feeling it much stronger when, after getting married, she moved to São Paulo City. She found the city very strange, she had no relatives there, she had very few friends and they lived far away, so she spent most of her time being alone. She only had her husband, but he had to work all day. In the house she felt nervous; she didn't manage to focus on anything, not even reading. Since her window was only a few meters away from the window of the neighbouring apartment and the sun hardly ever got into the house, she felt the space was suffocating and limited. When she went out, she found the city scary. She remembered a cold and cloudy day when she was walking down a street in her neighbourhood; she had a sensation of floating, her head dizzy, her hands sweating, feeling shaky and insecure – it occurred to her, that if 'something' would happen, she couldn't count on anybody. She was overwhelmed by panic. I asked her to draw this situation (Figure 10.3).

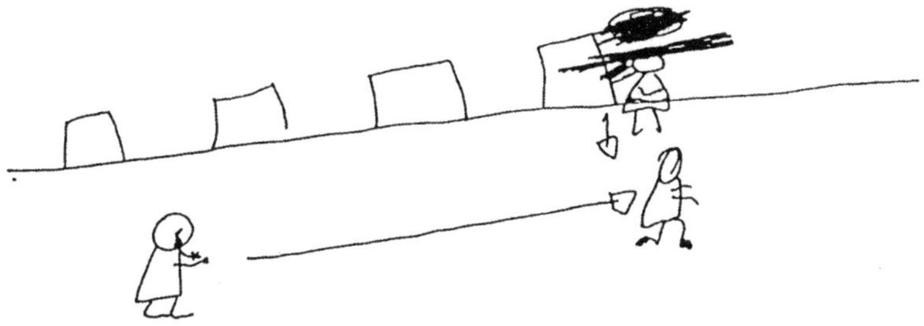

Figure 10.3 Martha walking down a street of her neighbourhood, a situation experienced with fear

Using the technique of 'concretization' again, I had a conversation with the symptom that Martha had drawn; investigating when was the first time that it had appeared in her life. I found out that she was six or seven years old. She was on the street walking home, being afraid of Zelao, a beggar who was dirty and used to walk around talking to himself. People used to say that he stole children. Young Martha suddenly noticed the he was sitting on the sidewalk. She got frightened and ran home. At night she dreamt of the beggar and woke up feeling scared, she started to cry and called for her mother. At this point I asked Martha to draw this scene (Figure 10.4). She drew the bedroom of her parents, who slept together with Martha's bed at their side.

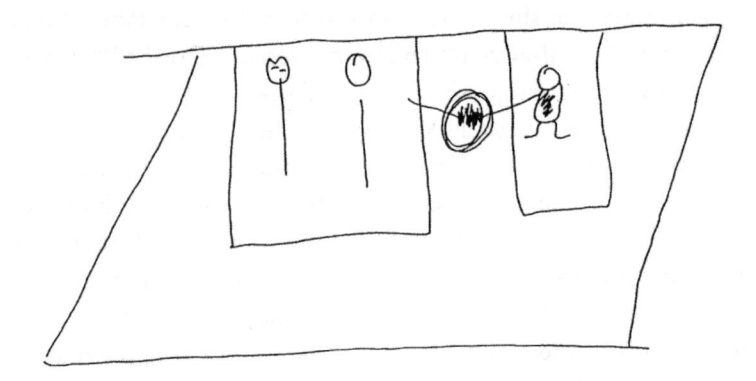

Figure 10.4 The bedroom where Martha slept with her parents in a protected situation

Here, I applied the technique of 'taking the role of the other' in order to investigate the internalized figures of the father and the mother and also to get further information regarding the situation in question.

I interviewed Martha in the roles of her father and mother. I found out from the father that Martha was his youngest child and that she was born premature; he had a lot of affection and fondness towards her. He also said that Martha still sleeps in the parents' bedroom because she is very fearful. From Martha's mother I found out that she is very attached to her daughter, they do nearly everything together and that Martha can only sleep if she is close to her.

In the soliloquy of her child-bed, Martha said that she had a bad dream; she dreamt that Zelao the beggar was running after her, she became scared and started to cry, calling for her mother. We continued describing the scene: the mother awoke and stretching her hand towards Martha's bed she started to caress the hand of her daughter. Little by little the child started to feel more relieved, calm and secure, eventually managing to go to sleep again.

Martha told me that she couldn't stay away from her mother, especially when she needed to sleep. When once invited by her cousins to go travel with them, even though she wished to go, she decided not to. The fear of sleeping far away from her mother prevented her from going; in some way this fear was also stimulated by the mother, who didn't like to be away from her daughter either.

This is how she was living in a small town. Her father was a distinguished person of the town, well known by everyone: Martha felt protected there. After getting married, she had to move to São Paulo, which was when her symptoms appeared.

At the end of the session Martha was talking more relaxed and calm, feeling freer. In the following sessions, she started to talk less and less about her symptoms and more and more about her life, about her difficulties and worries. At times, I used psychogram again, at other times we did dramatizations in which she managed to take part with gradually less and less fear. After some time, Martha started group psychotherapy.

Case example: Fabio

Fabio (a 22-year-old student) came to therapy with relationship difficulties. He was very shy, most of the time feeling embarrassed and flustered, thinking of himself as 'a boring guy' who has nothing to talk about; as a result he was very quiet. In groups he felt observed and embarrassed, blushing easily. His relationships were painful and distressing. In spite of being fond of people, he tended to isolate himself.

Fabio had been in group psychotherapy for some time, always being quiet, talking only when he was asked. In spite of finding it difficult to dramatize, he had been the protagonist a couple of times. He was very inhibited when playing roles, and usually preferred sessions that were exclusively verbal.

The session described in the following was attended by three clients. The session started with the group being silent, only asking about the other group members, who were still on their holidays. Then they asked for my working proposal. I suggested them to draw a life situation in which they experience worry or difficulty. The suggestion was accepted, so I distributed pens and paper, telling the clients that they had about half an hour to do the drawings. They finished much earlier, and Fabio was chosen by the group for work.

Fabio presented his drawing (Figure 10.5), explaining that he had tried to draw how he feels in front of groups (any group).
He told us that in front of groups he feels he is being observed by everybody. I asked him to 'concretize' this feeling on the drawing: a tight feeling in the throat, his heart beating fast, sweaty palms and a blush of the cheeks. He also

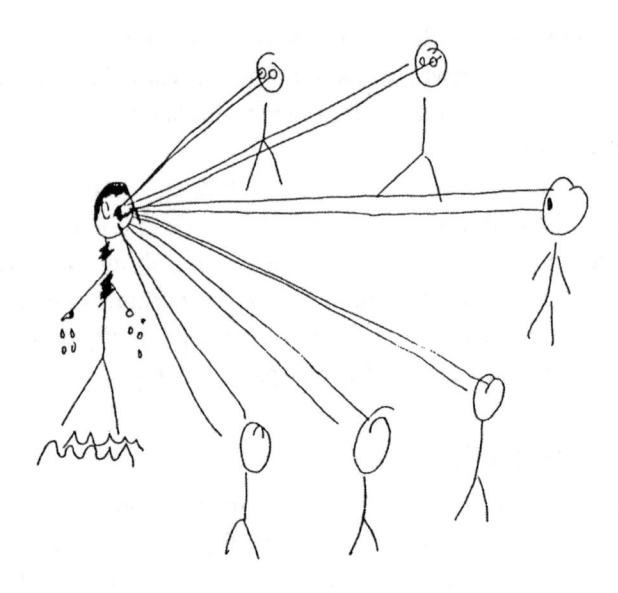

Figure 10.5 Fabio's drawing of how he feels in front of groups

described a floating feeling. In soliloquy he related feeling embarrassed, desperately trying to find an excuse to leave the situation.

I invited him to take on the role of one of his observers. In this role he said that Fabio was a quiet and shy person, but he was nice. I asked if there was anything else to say; the observer told me there wasn't, he didn't have any other information about Fabio. Following this, Fabio related that his internal feelings of discomfort are at times revealed by the blushing of his face.

We concretized the blushing and Fabio took on this role. In a conversation with the blush we found out that it appeared quite some years ago. I invited the blush to tell us an episode when it had appeared before. Fabio got out of role and told the group that once he fainted in the classroom. I asked him to draw this situation (Figure 10.6). It was a lesson about blood types, when each student had to determine his/her own blood type.

In the role of one of his class-mates, Fabio described himself as a good student and a good classmate. In the role of the demanding teacher, he described himself as a good and well-behaved student who accomplishes his obligations and duties.

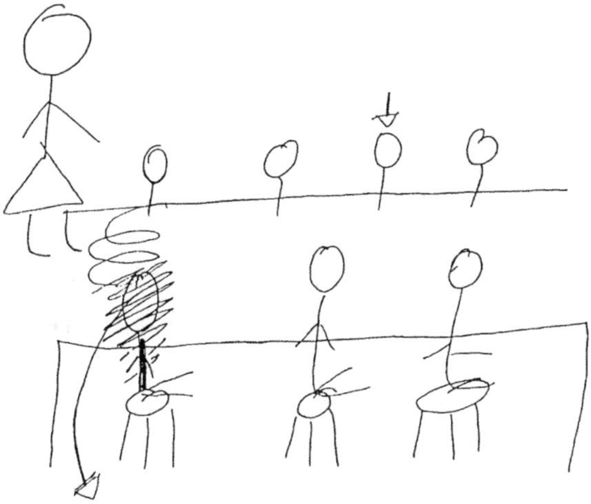

THE PSYCHOGRAM

Figure 10.6 Fabio's drawing of the classroom situation when he fainted

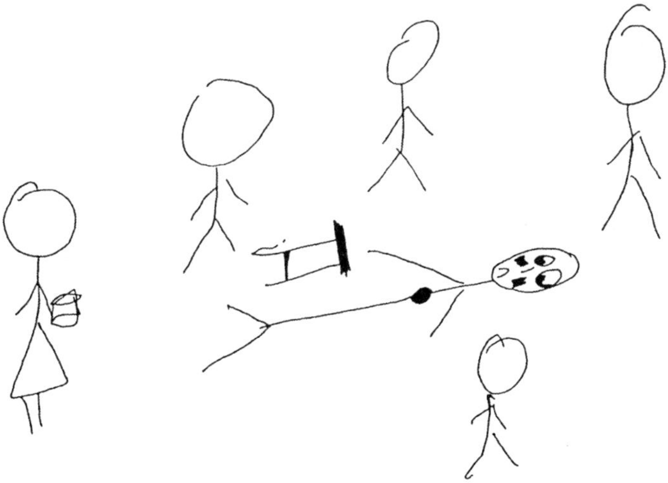

Figure 10.7 Fabio fallen to the floor, blushing and angry

In his own role Fabio related that every time he moved the needle towards his finger in order to collect the necessary blood-drops, he gave up. When he had finally managed to obtain the blood smear, everything darkened around him, and he started to feel dizzy. The next thing he remembered was being on the floor surrounded by his classmates and the teacher. I asked him to draw this scene (Figure 10.7).

The teacher (role taken by Fabio) related that she was frightened, because this had never happened before in any of her lessons. She brought sweetened water for Fabio. One of his classmates said that he didn't know Fabio had 'these things'. While lying on the floor, Fabio felt embarrassed and angry for what had happened. The blush appeared again, and so I invited Fabio to take on the role of the blush. We found out that it first appeared when Fabio was still a small child, and he 'peed in the bed'. Fabio remembered waking up wet one night, needing to go to his parents' bedroom to call his mother to change his pyjamas and sheets. At other times, his mother came to the bedroom and found him wet.

Fabio made a drawing of his bedroom (Figure 10.8) that he used to share with his younger brother. The mother is at the door, while Fabio is lying in bed wet and blushing. Taking on the role of his mother, she said that 'he is too old to pee in the bed'. Fabio otherwise would be an easy and good child, except the problem of his bedwetting.

Back in his own role, Fabio told how his mother had put a calendar on the wall, marking with a star all the days when he did not wet the bed. He felt very embarrassed when he 'did not deserve' the star. He also talked about the fear he experiences in situations which are out of his control and which disclose and reveal unpleasant aspects of him, thus putting his self-esteem at risk. Looking at his first drawing again, he smiled, thinking that his control to avoid surprises was excessive; it blocked him and made his relationships difficult and painful.

During this session, Fabio gained a deeper understanding of the reasons for his difficulties with relationships. Through the 'psychodramatic insight' (Bustos 1975) gained by this understanding he became more able to face his difficulties.

In the following I will briefly present one more drawing made by another group member in the same session.

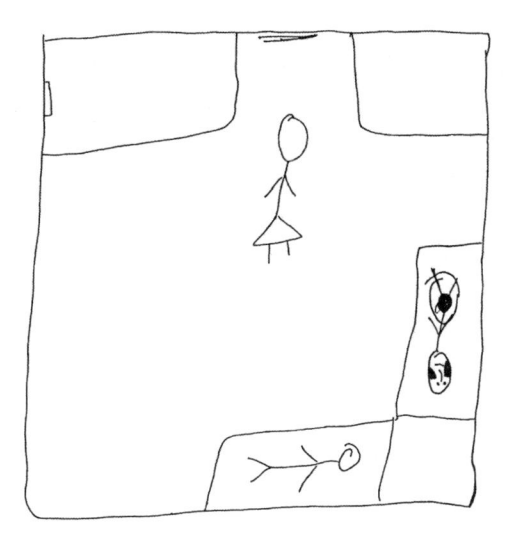

Figure 10.8 Fabio in his bed, wet and blushing. His mother has just entered the room; his brother is sleeping in the other bed

Case example: Lúcia

Lúcia divided the paper in four, in the first quarter drawing three people: her brother with his girlfriend and herself on the side. She explained that in spite of liking the other two, she didn't feel at ease with them. In the second quarter she drew herself on the side of her other brother and his girlfriend. Again, she had uneasy feelings being around them. In the third quarter Lúcia drew herself by the side of a woman called Vera (a member of the group); she had the same uneasy feeling in her presence. And finally, in the last quarter she drew herself and her mother, describing yet again the same feeling (Figure 10.9).

I asked her to take on the roles of each of the characters in the drawing. Lúcia was seen by the 'others' as a good, reserved, diligent and co-operative person; a good sister, good friend and good daughter.

I pointed out that in the two drawings on the top of the sheet she placed a man next to the women, while in the other two drawings she didn't. I asked her if she could complete these last two drawings. Since she looked hesitant at the third picture, I suggested that she drew the first person who comes to her mind. She drew me (the therapist) on Vera's side. With the last picture she was even more hesitant. I asked her whom could she place next to her mother, to which she responded that probably her father and her two brothers. Following this she started to tell about her competitive relationships with women and her difficulties in this competition. Most of the time she gave up, placing herself at the margin of these triangular relationships.

When, at the end of the session, I invited the group to share, they all seemed pleased. Fabio felt the session was helpful and was surprised by the amount of information he had gained from the drawings. Lúcia said that the session was interesting and it had helped her to see something that 'was so obvious'. Jose, the third member of the group made similarly positive comments. (Since the drawings of this third client would not directly serve the didactic objective of this chapter, I decided not to include them here.)

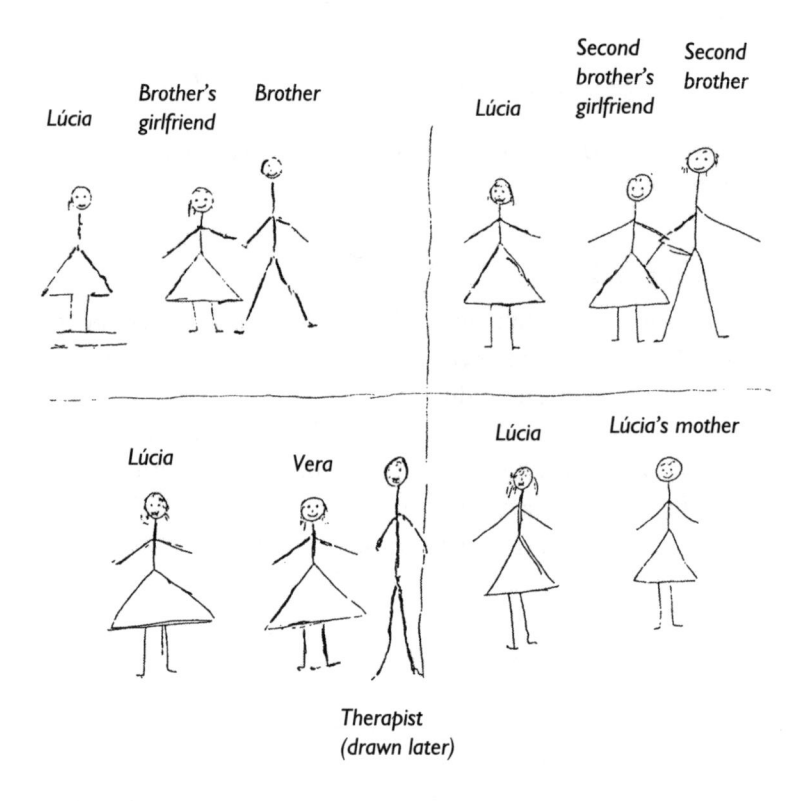

Figure 10.9 Lúcia's drawing depicting her in the presence of her two brothers and their girlfriends, Vera (another group member) and her mother.

Discussion

Psychogram is not a substitute for classical psychodrama. My intention when presenting it was more to describe it as a resource that can be used in psychodrama.

Psychogram differs from analytically oriented art therapy; in the latter, the patient is asked to produce a spontaneous piece of work, which is then discussed with the analyst, searching for the meaning of unconscious projections. These kinds of spontaneous productions are seen as a symbolic language. Analytical art therapy is based on the assumption that every individual (whether artistically trained or not) has the latent capacity to project his internal conflicts into images; through the graphic representation of these internal experiences, they will gain a better verbal articulation (Hammer 1978).

In the realm of psychology, drawings are also used in projective clinical tests as auxiliary methods to diagnosis (Buck's HTP test, Machover's test of drawing two people, etc.). Among other arguments, these tests are based on the assumption that creative productions reveal the individual's needs more directly than any other kind of activity. In order to use drawing as a projective test, the process needs to be standardized. During the interpretation of these tests the following aspects can be taken into consideration: the size and symmetry of the drawing, the pressing of the pencil against the paper, the type of lines used, the details and the content of the drawing, etc. (Hammer 1978).

The use of the psychogram doesn't need to be standardized. The drawings consist of graphically represented scenes of the protagonist's internal world; interpretation is done concomitantly while the pictures are drawn. Components of any drawing can be transformed into roles to be performed; the objective of this role play is a better understanding of the material in focus. This can be stimulating for the patient, who will feel more responsible for his own therapeutic process. This effect is more visible when using psychogram with adolescents.

According to Naumburg (in Hammer 1978), drawings can liberate deeper unconscious material quicker and therefore can speed up the therapeutic process. He explains this with the fact that instead of words, internal experiences are translated mainly into images. According to Hammer (1978), drawings can be seen as a mirror placed in front of the internal constitution (character) of the person, reflecting the different aspects of his personality and the equilibrium between these.

Freud (1977, p.113) wrote that: 'Part of the difficulty of supplying a description of dreams is due to our limitation in translating these images into words; I could draw it – the dreamer often tells us – but I don't know how to do it.' Freud believed that the unconscious communicates through images, but interestingly he did not use drawings in his therapeutic work. An account given in the form of a drawing can be richer than a verbal account.

The psychotherapeutic method at times follows the presentation of the past, re-living step-by-step the conflict that worries us in a given moment (Bustos 1975). In his 'Study of Hysteria' Freud wrote that hysteric syndromes can disappear when we manage to awake (revive) the memory and the concomitant affective state of the process that provoked these symptoms. According to Jaspers (1979), simply knowing, meditating or pondering over the past cannot lead to any therapeutic effect; in order to achieve this effect the past needs to be re-lived. With his proposal of psychodrama, Moreno goes even further when stating that psychodramatic treatment consists in inducing in the subject an adequate representation of the dimensions of his private world.

At the core of psychodrama is dramatization; however, since action can also manifest itself in other ways (words, drawings, etc.), psychodrama shouldn't limit itself only to dramatization. According to Bustos (1975, pp.61-2):

> our work consists in choosing the way of communication that represents the richest potential in a given moment. If we lose the words, we need to move to the action; if the action becomes inexpressive, we'll only take the movement. We always need to find that remnant aspect of communication which is infiltrated with the truth. It is the therapist's mission to recognize this aspect and make use of it.

When classic dramatic action and words only generate resistance, the psychogram can contribute to the lessening of this ressistance.

Blatner (1969/70) writes that in our culture there is a tendency to distrust action and emotion. The externaliztion and showing of emotions are seen as artificial, being connected to the theatre and conceived as frivolous and unreal. This can lead to the fear of losing control in the psychodramatic action. By using drawings (and thus reducing the need for vigilance) this fear can be attenuated, resistance can be diminished, and issues can emerge much easier.

Working with groups of children, Moccio and Córdoba (in Martinez Bouquet, Moccio and Pavlovsky 1975) used dramatic techniques in the elaboration of drawings. Their objective was to allow the emergence of unconscious material in a shorter time (compared to other known techniques) and to liberate children from conventional and stereotypical images that may impede the emergence of more authentic and spontaneous ones.

According to the testimony of clients with whom I used the psychogram, this technique has proved successful in facilitating therapeutic communication, by making their reports (of a problematic situation) more focused and the analysis more objective. Psychogram was also perceived as a pleasant and enjoyable way of undertaking therapeutic work. I also had the experience of the clients themselves asking for the use of drawings.

When working with drawings, sessions generally have a more relaxed atmosphere, without diminishing the emotional level. Communication between therapist and client becomes easier and flowing. The attention of the group members doesn't dilute, on the contrary, it becomes more focused on what is developing from the drawing. In terms of Rojas-Bermudez's (1985) 'role structure' (see chapter 5), roles emerge much more easily. Since the boundary of the self does not expand, the majority the individual's roles are accessible (they can be performed). There are certain similarities between the psychogram and Rojas-Bermudez's concept of the 'intermediary object'; however, since drawings do not fulfil all the characteristics described by Rojas-Bermudez (1985), they cannot be considered as 'intermediary object'. Bermudez described the following eight characteristics (of the intermediary object) as necessary:

1. Real and concrete existence.
2. Harmless: it doesn't unchain an alarm reaction.
3. Malleability: it can be easily used in any role-play involving complementary roles.
4. Transmissibility: it is a mediator of communication, a substitute for the therapist–patient link, while it maintains the distance between the two people.
5. Adaptability: it adapts to the needs of the client.
6. Assimilability: it allows such an intimate relationship, that the client can identify with the intermediary object.
7. Instrumentality: it can be used as an extension of the client.
8. Identificability: it can be recognized immediately.

As we have seen, the psychogram doesn't fulfil all of these characteristics. Drawing is an instrument that only starts to exist from the moment it was created. I would like to stress the difference between the psychogram and the intermediary object regarding transmissibility: when using the psychogram, communication doesn't happen through the drawing itself, but it is a direct communication between therapist and protagonist; and in no way does the drawing substitute the link – on the contrary, it is trying to facilitate it.

Drawings also often serve as a warm-up for a proper dramatization that may lead to a catharsis of integration. According to Moreno (1974) it is the 'catharsis of integration' that gives a real therapeutic feeling to psychodrama. I believe that the psychogram promotes and fosters 'psychodramatic insight', that is, a deep and emotional perception of a previously obscure situation (Bustos 1975).

As with classical dramatization, dramatization through drawings can be used with any person or any situation. The use of the psychogram is more strongly indicated in cases when classical dramatization cannot be applied. Classical dramatization may be problematic due to external factors (for example, lack of space) or due to factors related to the client (for example, a limiting physical condition, or a blockage of spontaneity that manifests itself in the limitation of the corporal action). I also use the psychogram when there is a risk of 'irrational acting-out' during a traditional dramatization (for example, in case of patients who cannot control their impulsivity). This technique has been used successfully with psychotic patients who have productive symptoms, such as deliriums and hallucinations. The concretization of these symptoms in drawings may help their understanding and, therefore, their therapeutic handling.

I would also like to propose the application of the psychogram for the investigation of the social atom, mainly in the case of adolescents. When working with this objective, I ask the adolescents to make a drawing of their family in a scene (which they can choose); then, through role-taking, we start to investigate the roles involved. At times, this alone can bring therapeutic results.

I have never submitted a client only to the use of psychogram over the therapeutic process; I always used a blend of psychogram and classical dramatization in ongoing psychotherapy.

My intention within this chapter was to explain this technique, and by making it public, hopefully encourage some more in-depths discussions regarding its use.

Note

1   Originally published under the title: 'Psicograma: utilização do desenho em psicoterapia psicodramática'. *TEMAS Journal 21*, pp.101–127, 1981, São Paulo.

11

Genodrama
Psychodramatic work with genograms in couple therapy[1]

Maria Amalia Faller Vitale

> Marriage or the union of two people is surrounded by a powerful halo of choices, options and freedom; however, it is clear that this union is also strongly connected and anchored to something that reaches beyond these choices, something in which not the individual is the driving force or focal point. (Velho 1986)

When trying to reflect on contemporary marital liaisons, we realize that the concepts of couple and family are strongly interconnected. Even if the forms of living in a marital relationship are changing, the criteria for choosing partners remain the same. These criteria are delineated by affective and sexual references and are marked by familial, socio-economic and cultural conditions. Therefore, the forming of a couple presupposes mutual choices at both a conscious and unconscious level.[2] As Munhoz (2000) points out (in his study of reproduced and discontinued family patterns), a matrimonial bond doesn't just simply refer to the relationship between two individuals, but it also includes the internalized relational network of both partners. During the different stages of the family life-cycle, the members of a couple tend to involve themselves (to different degrees) with their family networks.

Within the sociometric network of the family we can distinguish two dimensions: a horizontal dimension (consisting of links of the same level, that is, relationships within the same generation – sisters, brothers, sisters-in-law, etc.) and another, vertical or inter-generational dimension (consisting of inter-generational links – grandparents–parents–children).[3] The marital relationship may have more or less autonomy in relation to this network. This will also result in a certain degree of tension.

The thoughts and reflections that are going to be presented in this chapter are based on the recognition of the importance of this sociometric family network, and are the result of my clinical work (with families and couples) focusing on the cross-generational transmission of the 'family world'(Vitale 1994).[4]

When working with couple therapy, it is impossible to avoid the issue of family transmission, not only in the trans-generational or inter-generational sense, but also in the sense of the interconnectedness of the partners' symbolical inheritance that they receive and/or transform. My experience within this field of work has shown that although couples create new references, at the same time they do not abandon the old references of their primary family identity. It is also important to remember that the process of re-adaptation to the transmitted legacies and inheritances doesn't occur in a linear way, neither on the level of the individual or the level of the couple.

Therefore, the patterns (history) of the primary family are integrated (in different degrees) into the relational heritage of a couple; in the therapeutic process, these can be understood through the means of genodrama.

The genogram

The objective of this chapter is to present the use of genodrama in couple and family therapy, that is, to focus on the psychodramatic potential of the genogram – an instrument acknowledged by family therapists. The genogram is a clinical tool that can help us understand couples and families through the prism of the transmission process of family life.

The genogram is not just the simple graphic representation of the paternal and maternal family genealogy; the genogram also provides us with information about the family members and their relationships within at least three generations. It helps us form a quick gestalt of the family network and of the basic family patterns that developed and inter-crossed over the years. It marks the main stages of the family life-cycle (McGoldrick and Gerson 1985).

A genogram will provide information that is more general (for example, names and dates of significant events), as well as more complex information, such as repetitive relationship patterns (for example, triangular relationships). The information obtained through this diagram will serve as a source of therapeutic hypotheses. As a result, the clinical problems presented by the symptomatic family member can more easily be related to the family context.

Those who work with families and couples know that genograms demonstrate the trans-generational passing down of family-related traditions; they also reveal those specific family beliefs and behaviours that promote (influence) the individualization process of the family members (Sampaio and Gameiro 1985). Because it provides a tangible form for the representation of the family, the genogram has been widely used in the clinical field. Based on the genogram, a subjective interpretation of the family history can be obtained.

Many therapists use the genogram in the first session of a therapy process, revising it when new information arises. When used in the initial interview, the genogram may also help to involve the family members in the therapy process (McGoldrick and Gerson 1985). As I already mentioned, through the means of this instrument the family tends to visualize the current problems within the family group; the therapist and the family gather a wide range of information regarding the family life and the family's structure on the generational level. This will bring an understanding of the family in time and space, as well as in its horizontal and vertical dimension. The genogram facilitates the formulation of questions regarding the relationship patterns developed and repeated within the family. The genogram is usually prepared within a therapy session, together with the family; the potential gaps in the genogram can be filled in with the information gathered during the later stages of the therapy process. We can distinguish between simple and more complex genograms. These latter can portray families with numerous divorces and re-marriages over the generations.

Approaching the genogram from a systemic and relational perspective, McGoldrick and Gerson (1985) have distinguished the following categories for the analysis of the genogram: the family structure; patterns through the life cycle; repetitive patterns between the generations; life events and family functioning; relational patterns and triangles; stable and unstable families. (Unfortunately though, the physical limitations of this chapter do not allow me to discuss all these categories in detail.)

The origins of the genogram are related to those family therapy models that use a multi-generational perspective. Today however, it is used by various family therapists working with different approaches. Those who support Bowen's (1978) approach, use the genogram as a *primary* instrument to access the family. During their training, family therapists are often required to construct and interpret their own genogram, in order to improve their relationships with their own primary families and to better develop their professional role as therapists. This also explains why many family therapists (with different orientations and backgrounds) have been reflecting on the use of the genogram.[5] More recently, the genogram has also been used as a tool for research.[6]

Let us now look at how a psychodrama family therapist works with the genogram.

Psychodramatic work with couples

In order to present my psychodramatic work developed from the use of the genogram, it is necessary to first review some of Moreno's contributions to family therapy. Even though these contributions were precursory, there was very little recognition of them within the movement of family therapy. I would like to highlight that the perspective developed by the systemic approach (which constitutes the foundations of family therapy) was already present in Moreno's contributions. In a paper establishing the correlations between psychodrama and the systems theory, Seixas (1992) has shown us that some of the systemic principles are present in Moreno's work.

Since he focused his attention on the interrelations of the people forming a group, we can consider Moreno as a forerunner of systems-centred therapists. Clearly, Moreno's ideas represent a shift in the *locus* of therapy. He started to look at the family as a conjunction between parents and children, between husband and wife. However, as I mentioned above, Moreno wasn't duly recognized in the history of family therapy.

Let us have a brief overview of Moreno's ideas relevant to family therapy. His pioneering approach is evident as much in his ideas, as in his practise. He worked with families from the beginning of his career:

> Moreno often helped families in difficulty by discussing their problems and possible solutions openly with them, repeating his experience with the prostitutes in Vienna. He called this spontaneous approach *théatre reciproque* [reciprocal theatre]. ... *Théatre reciproque* is based on systems theory and is an ancestor of family and community therapy. (Marineau 1989, pp.68-69)

In 1921 Moreno founded the Theatre of Spontaneity, and through the means of dramatizations worked with the Barbara case.[7] Thus Moreno had created the basis of the psychodramatic therapeutic action for couples (that was further developed later on). In *Who shall survive?* (1934) Moreno developed the theoretical postulates of socio-dynamics that formed the basis for the study of groups (such as the family). In the focus of socio-dynamics is the individual, within his/her relational configurations such as dyads, triangles, circles, sociometric networks, social atoms – these being governed by the forces of attraction, rejection and neutrality. These configurations can be captured by the sociometric tests and mapped by the sociograms.

Moreno's first psychodramatic treatment of a couple was in 1939, in the Therapeutic Theatre (Beacon, New York). Moreno worked in separate sessions with the husband, the wife and the husband's lover. Pavlovsky notes the following regarding the case:

> In an article entitled 'The Psychodrama of a Marriage', Moreno describes a passionate literary report of the vicissitudes of three classical protagonists in a marital drama. Their treatment lasted for ten sessions, with regular weekly intervals. The richness of this historical treatment enabled Moreno to treat simultaneously the three protagonists of this conflict. (Martinez Bouquet *et al.* 1975, p.53)

Moreno himself described this work, as a situation which was painful on the one hand, but on the other led to results by bringing together the three participants to a direct confrontation and by helping (within the therapeutic context) to clarify the conjugal conflict. Moreno also points out that his attendance to these three protagonists impeded a possible suicide attempt of one of them. '…the separation of the couple and the dispersion of the affair have given the three of them the chance for a new start. The knot was disentangled' (Moreno 1974, p.215).

Moreno's ideas converging towards a relational perspective were presented in 1946, in his book *Psychodrama, Vol.1*, and later on in *Psychodrama, Vols. 2 and 3*.

In a clear way, Moreno states that working with couples: 'appeared to revolutionize all customary concepts of psychiatric treatment. I recognized that in a truly inter-personal neurosis, this neurosis exists only as long as a controversial flow of emotions between two persons exists' (Moreno 1946, p.236).

Thus, in Moreno's view:

> Marriage and family therapy has to be so conducted that the 'interpsyche' of the entire group is re-enacted so that their tele relations, their co-conscious and co-unconscious states are brought to life. Co-conscious and co-unconscious states, are by definition, such states which the partners have experienced and produced jointly and which

can, therefore, be only jointly reproduced or re-enacted. (Moreno 1946, p.vii)

From this perspective, the therapeutic agent is not the single person, but the family group. This relational dimension emerges in all the main Morenian concepts.

Moreno analyses the cases of conjugal conflicts, through the prism of the social and role atoms, that is, in terms of satisfying and unsatisfying roles. In this respect, the roles have a systemic nature (Williams 1989). In this sense, in order to be concretized, a role demands an interpersonal experience, and therefore the involvement of two or more individuals. Together with the concepts of role, social atom[8] and cultural atom, Moreno also developed diagrams representing the individual's and the community's social atom. These diagrams are interpreted in terms of the tele-structure.[9]

Moreno (1974) presents the social atom of a psychotic universe, describing the dramatic way of 'undoing' and 'rebuilding' the social configuration of interpersonal relationships of a psychotic patient, illustrating this case with socigrams. Through the sociograms he portrays the distribution and intensity of tele within the various social atoms.

When he introduced the psychodramatic method in Switzerland, Moreno (1974) made references to Friedemann's[10] 'atogram'. This was a modification of Moreno's action diagram,[11] which combined with the sociogram, resulted in a highly valuable diagnostic method. These diagrams (as graphic representations) have some similarities with the genogram, in the sense that they gather information referring to the horizontal dimension of the family group and that they mark the distribution of the tele relationships.

It is also interesting to recall that, based on Moreno's reflections and thoughts, Schutzenberger (1997) uses the term geno-sociogram to describe the instrument which:

> allows a sociometric representation, based on the family tree. ...The geno-sociogram is the commented representation of the family tree (genogram), highlighting the sociometric links and relationships of the individual as well as his/her involvement with the different people and different relationships: co-presence, pairs, triangles, exclusions, etc. (Schutzenberger 1997, pp.19–20)

Since, within the realm of family sociodrama, a consistent theoretical body still hasn't been reached, exploring the advantages and potentials of action methods within the family therapy continues to represent a challenge.

Moreno told us that there are many action methods, and that therapists can create and re-create them in accordance with the new necessities: 'When a new necessity arises, therapists frequently find themselves obliged to create a new method, or to modify an older one, in order to resolve the difficulties of a given situation' (Moreno 1974, p.130). In another paragraph, while describing the psychodramatic method, Moreno (1974, p.118) states: 'the use of the psychodramatic method is practically unlimited. However, the nucleus of the method remains unchanged.'

Thus my experimenting with the application of the genogram and other action techniques were anchored in the Morenian contributions, stimulated by the challenges of working with couples and persuaded by the necessity of discovering creative ways of exploring family relationships. Dramatizing the different aspects of the genogram has proved to be a fertile resource for penetrating the core of family relationships. I denominated this kind of work as genodrama.

The genodrama

Genodrama can be used in various stages of couple or family therapy; there are many possibilities within the therapeutic process for its application. In the case of every couple there is a stage of the therapeutic process when the use of genodrama is appropriate or possible, however, there is no strict rule regarding when to apply it.

My objective when working with the genogram has been to investigate the relational patterns that repeat themselves or are modified within the different generations. It also allows for both members of the couple to find their own place within their primary families and their path of individualization. While maintaining the focus presented by the couple, this technique facilitates the recognition of each member of the conjugal relationship. The more specific aim of the genogram is to capture the movements of re-organization of the family guidelines along the generations, and their re-interpretations by the protagonists themselves.

In order to present the psychodramatic potential of the genogram, in the following I will exemplify its use through a clinical case.

I start the work by introducing the different symbols used in the genogram to the couple. I give a general explanation regarding how to construct a genogram, addressing the doubts that may arise. After constructing the genogram – this being done during a therapeutic session – I ask the couple to mark all the significant information related to the genogram. (I usually work with the above presented categories by McGoldrick and Gerson [1985], expanding on these with others that I have developed over the years.) My experience is that couples and families usually construct their genograms with spontaneity, and often in a playful atmosphere. Based on the genogram, I move on to the psychodramatic work, that is, genodrama.

Case example: Maria and Paulo

A couple came to therapy with the complaint that their marriage had become difficult after the birth of their first child. 'We do not manage to talk; our arguments get increasingly worse; we even thought about separating.' The couple spent quite a few years trying to have a baby. They have been married for eight years, and they have a 9-month-old child. Maria, the wife, is 33; she is an occupational therapist. Paulo, the husband is 34; he is an architect.

They reveal a certain sense of guilt for relating their arguments to the birth of their daughter. Their discussions involved complaints and mutual accusations. They also told me, that following Maria's return to work,[12] both of their mothers had started helping to look after the baby. As a result, the couple has more proximity to the family network. This closeness (to the family network) was also a reason for their increased mutual dissatisfaction.

I pursued the possibility that part of the couple's complaints was related to the adaptation to the changes in the family life-cycle and to the form of participation in the family network. Taking this context into consideration, I invited both members of the couple to construct their genogram. I pointed out various aspects that could be observed in the genogram along the generations. I asked them to notice all the aspects that are repetitive and to note all the information which they considered important. First, they both constructed their own genograms. Following this, I invited them to exchange their genograms and to discuss every observation regarding their own and their partner's genogram.

Following this, I invited the partners to return to their own genograms, and internally to ask themselves what came to their attention and what caused feelings of tension in them while they were talking and listening to the other. I also asked them to identify any possible doubts regarding the genogram (on either the horizontal or vertical level), and to notice the predominant feeling while having this internal conversation. With this warm-up, the path to the following dramatziation was also delineated.

Maria relates that she felt the presence of her grandmothers very intensely, even though they had both died when she was still an adolescent (one five years after the other). She had been closer to her maternal grandmother.

Paulo tells us that while constructing his genogram, he became disappointed by how little he knew about his paternal family (his parents separated when he was still a child). Paulo's father returned to the country of his origin. His contacts with his father and paternal family were thus very haphazard and occasional. However, he remembered his grandfather, whom he met when visiting his father.

Maria's genodrama

I suggested to Maria that she concentrate on her own genogram (Figure 11.1) and to visualize her grandmothers, as they were on photographs. I asked her to select one of her internal photographs. Following this, I used *relationship psychotherapy*, a technique developed by Fonseca (2004), derived from classical psychodrama. A role play took place between the protagonist and her internalized grandmothers (their roles were taken on and role reversals were done by Maria and the therapist). All this time her husband observed, and then was invited to share. Through this psychodramatic process, we explored the legacies and beliefs of Maria's family, as well as the different roles and positions held by the women within this family.

In the role of her maternal grandmother, the protagonist made the following statement: 'A woman should know how to sacrifice herself for her family, and should understand the lapses of men, because marriage and family are the most important things in the life of a woman.' While in this role, the protagonist took on the physical posture of a depressed and solitary figure. In the role of her paternal grandmother, she said: 'A woman shouldn't be foolish; she should know how to deal with her husband!' The body posture of the paternal grandmother was erect and assertive.

Maria recognized that within her family there were contradictory views regarding the situation of women. Next, she brought forth the figure of her mother. Taking on her role, she revealed a sad and solitary person. In the roles of the three women – Maria's grandmothers and her mother – the strong generational ties that occur among the women of her family could be observed. Her father appeared as being excluded from this female network, but at the same time he also authorized it.

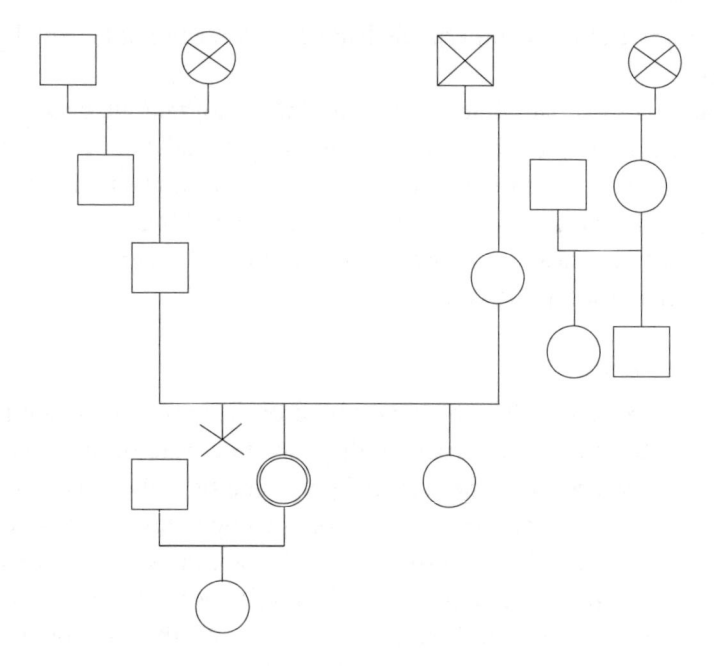

Figure 11.1 Maria's genogram. Key to symbols: ☐ *man;* ○ *woman;* Ⓞ *client (Maria);* ☒ *deceased man;* ⊗ *deceased woman;* ✕ *induced abortions;* ⊔ *marriage*

Paulo's genodrama

As mentioned above, Paulo displayed a certain curiosity towards the paternal side of his family. I invited him to visualize his genogram (Figure 11.2) and to get in touch with his predominant feelings and sensations. The image of his paternal grandfather emerged, and similarly to Maria, I used relationship psychotherapy again. Paulo presented his grandfather as 'a strong and determined character in relation to life'. Through successive role reversals, Paulo's anger towards his father came to the surface. Paulo blamed his father for abandoning him. He asked his grandfather to (symbolically) pass on to him the masculine inheritance of the family, which he had not received (from his father). He described these male family legacies as necessary for him to be a man and a father. He had difficulties playing the role of the father. This role play helped the protagonist bring to the surface his feelings regarding family life. Paulo also related that he was resentful towards his mother, blaming her for the fact that his father left. His family experiences were marked by

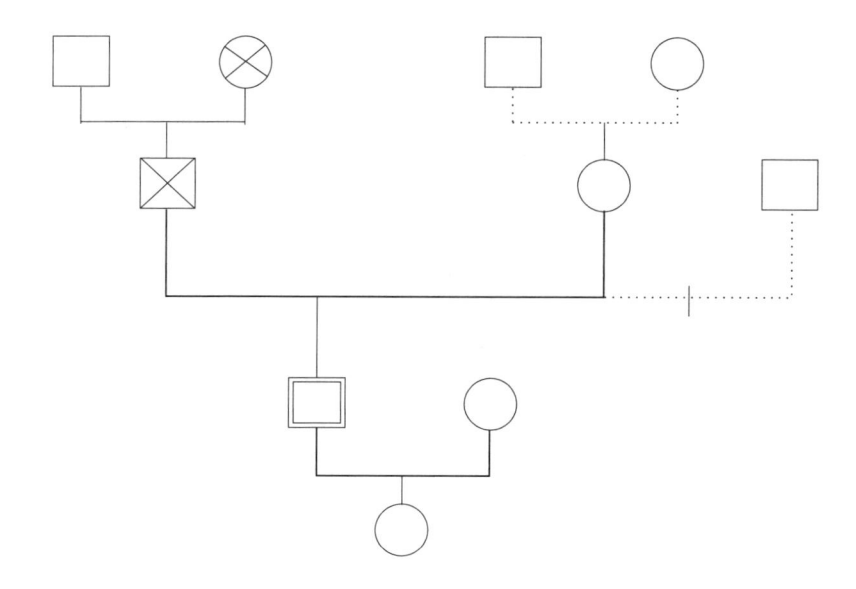

Figure 11.2 Paulo's genogram. Key to symbols: ☐ *man;* ○ *woman;* ☐ *client (Paulo);* ⊠ *deceased man;* ⊗ *deceased woman;* ⌐⌐ *marriage;* ⌐⌐ *separation;* ⌐⌐ *couple living together without being legally married*

feminine relationships Paulo lived with his mother in the house of his maternal grandmother a single mother too .

After the psychodramatic work, the couple shared their impressions. Thus, in light of this process, the relational focus presented by the couple was re-directed.

Reflections

Paulo expresses both fear and fascination for the female alliances which he had lived together with throughout his life mother grandmother, wife daughter . He is afraid of not being able to get close to his daughter. He is resentful for the lack of a *father model*. His wife's more active posture towards their daughter just further confirms his sense of failure as a father. Paulo says that Maria's understanding attitude also a characteristic of Maria's maternal grandmother was one of those personality traits that attracted him most towards her. Today, however, the psychological traits of her paternal grandmother authoritarianism and hardness are the most outstanding.

From Maria's perspective, both of the ambiguous 'feminine' legacies (that she received) reveal a male figure that is fragile in front of women; either because this fragile figure needs to be socially and emotionally 'supported', or because it needs to be 'neutralized'.

The birth of their daughter precipitated in the couple's relationship roles that were underdeveloped or concealed. Genodrama helped them both to get in touch with the relational plot of their families built up over the generations. Even though they apparently already knew each other's family stories, playing the roles of their internalized family figures enabled the couple to see themselves and the other from a new angle. The couple had the chance to capture important complementary aspects of their relationship. These aspects constitute exteriorizations of the co-conscious and co-unconscious states experienced by the couple.

The role play was eventually broadened to such an extent that the partners played the roles of each other's ancestors – the objective of this was to develop spontaneity in the marital relationship. (For example, Maria's grandmother and Paulo's grandfather had a conversation. This change of context enabled the couple to re-create their own dialogue.) They also carried out interviews with the characters of their families, this allowing them to rebuild the plot of their relational patterns.

These fragments of dramatic work with the genogram clearly reveal how in response to a new phase of the family life-cycle (the presence of a new family member), the conflicts and beliefs constructed over the generations of the protagonists' families can re-emerge. The expectations, emotions and feelings contained within these family beliefs, reverberate in the marital drama. Thus, genodrama has the potential to unveil the transmission and transition processes within the world of the family. Through the demystification of the family histories, subtle mechanisms are revealed at the inter-generational level, which will broaden the realm of therapeutic possibilities. As Moreno pointed it out, 'role-play can be used as a method to explore unknown worlds and to expand the self' (Moreno 1974, p.220).

Genodrama can be used with either of the partners within one or more sessions. However, during the psychodramatic work other aspects may also arise, and new information may come to the surface during the therapy; these will allow the couple to re-visit their family histories and to re-write the script of their drama.

I would like to point out that when working with genodrama (either in couple therapy or workshops for professionals trained in family therapy) it is common for the figures of the grandparents to emerge. Clients often relate that they didn't imagine that grandparents can have such a powerful (latent) influence on their adult life. During discussions and role plays, grandparents appear as the mouthpiece (spokesmen) of the family. This leads us to the following two points of reflection: firstly, genogram and genodrama is an instrument that intrinsically facilitates the tri-and trans-generational dimension; and secondly, grandparents have an important role or symbolic function within the family network. Regarding this second point, some authors, such as Dolto (1992), noted the symbolic value that grandparents play in the structuring of the models with which children identify; their value as sources of transmission of the family history. Grandparents also play an important role in the re-drawing of the current family boundaries (Vitale 2003).

Obviously, there are many other aspects that could be explored when working with the genogram. My intention, however, was to offer a new context for working with couples and families, a new and creative technique that would help couples move on from their repetitive discussions. Both psychodramatists and systemic therapists tend to see the crystallization (rigidity) of family relationships as the lack of spontaneity:

> Family sociodrama appeals to spontaneity in order to enable families re-create their relationships. It aims to challenge the existing set of rules (which are often hidden) and to find new alternatives in front of the changes within the family structure. A therapeutic approach that is based on the principle of spontaneity will use dramatic action as well as verbal interventions; it aims to free up the energies blocked because of feelings of guilt, invisible loyalties and alliances; it offers a possibility for the family group to recognize their challenges in front of the changes that occurred in its life cycle. (Vitale 1999, p.177)

In each stage of the family life cycle, certain states of intergenerational relationships, as well as movements of increasing proximity or distancing (rupture) from these relationships (network) will emerge. In this respect, the current complaints of a couple can be contextualized within the time-span of the family.

The use of genodrama enables couples to recover the context, recreate the past, to open up a space for the future, and to re-weave the fabric of invisible loyalties in which the partners are imprisoned and caught up at the present.

By applying the genogram technique, important and significant information can be gathered, opening up innumerable possibilities for the dramatic work. Within the dramatic context, genodrama allows the emergence of the sociometric family network, representing all its various generational levels. Beyond the dramatization of the genogram and the role-play, other techniques (such as double and soliloquy) can also be used in this therapeutic situation that involves the couple and the therapist.

In conclusion, I would like to emphasize that as a sociodramatist, I do not look at the genealogical perspective (and thus genodrama) as merely a diagnostic tool of the family pathology; I see it more as a technique that allows the members of a couple or family to converge in a single social family history.

Notes

1 Originally published under the title: 'Genodrama: trabalho psicodramático com genograma em terapia de casal'. In M.A.F. Vitale, (ed) (2004) *Laços Amorosos – Terapia de Casal e Psicodrama [Love Relationships – Couple Therapy and Psychodrama]*, pp.233–251, São Paulo: Ágora.

2 For more details see Willi (1978), Berenstein (1990) and Munhoz (2000). According to Munhoz, when choosing partners, people are also strongly influenced by the patterns of their own primary families, either in the sense that they try to continue the family history, or that they try to break away from it. In other words, these choices have the tendency either to reproduce or to discontinue the family pattern.

3 Angelo (1995) used the term 'trigenerational', however, I prefer the term 'intergenerational', because in my view it describes better the idea of generational interchange.

4 Relations between generations and gender relationships are interconnected. In psychoanalysis, paternal and maternal transmissions are considered equally important in the unconscious heritage of the individual; these transmissions are also differentiated within the psychic structure of the individual.

5 Groisman, Lobo and Cavour (1996) for example, used the genogram to study the family mission.

6 Marques (2001) used the genogram (together with other instruments) in a generational research of working children.

7 As it is known by psychodramatists, the Barbara case marks the transformation of the spontaneous theatre into the Therapeutic Theatre, and later into Psychodrama. Barbara was an actress performing ingenuous and romantic roles: she married a

poet, a frequent spectator of her performances. Moreno was approached by the husband some time later, with certain complaints about Barbara: at home she was the opposite of her roles; rude and often physically aggressive. Moreno developed a dramatic action in order to help her change her attitudes towards her husband and eventually also introduced this approach in treatment.

8   The social atom refers to the relational network in which the individual is involved (inserted), taking into consideration the different social configurations to which the individual belongs (for example, family, friends, work, etc.).

9   Moreno defined tele as something that: 'grows out of person-to-person or person-to-object contacts from the birth level on and gradually develops the sense for inter-personal [social] relationships. ...It is an experience of some real factor in the other person's situation' (Moreno 1946, pp.238–239). Tele is based on reciprocity, and not just attraction (*positive tele*) or rejection (*negative tele*). It consists in the perception of the other and of the self within a situation. For Moreno, tele represents the basis of all healthy interrelationships and it is the foundation of all forms of psychotherapy.

10 According to Moreno (1974), 'Friedemann was the first European psychiatrist who, in 1926, used psychodramatic methods with psychiatric clients.'

11 This concept was used by Moreno himself (1974, p.130), but I have not found any further references to it.

12 In Brazil maternity leave is only three months.

12

Dramatic multiplication[1]

Pedro Mascarenhas

This chapter is based on my dissertation (Mascarenhas 1995), presented for the accreditation of becoming a psychodrama trainer-supervisor with the Brazilian Psychodrama Federation. My intention is to present the historical background and the definition of the concept of 'dramatic multiplication', as well as indications for its practical applications.

Historical background

The concept of dramatic multiplication was first outlined in the 1970s by Pavlovsky, Kesselman and Frydlewsky (1978) in their book published in Buenos Aires entitled: *Scenes Feared by Group Facilitators*. Between 1978 and 1980 Kesselman and Pavlovsky continued working in Madrid and Gothenburg with group didactic analysis (their work was presented in the article entitled 'Group didactic analysis' [1980]), while Frydlewsky further developed this concept in Buenos Aires. Already in 1974, in an article entitled 'The personality of the psychotherapist', Pavlovsky (1974, p.88) had made some precursory references to the concept of dramatic multiplication. During the 1980s their investigation continued with research around the creative matrix, presented in the book *Space and Creativity* (Pavlovsky 1980).

In 1982, Wilson Castello de Almeida made reference to the correlation between Umberto Eco's 'Open composition' (1991) and psychodrama (Almeida 1982, p.123).

In 1987, Kesselman, Pavlovsky and Frydlewsky published an article entitled 'The open composition of Umberto Eco and dramatic multiplication', in which they stated clearly and explicitly for the first time what they meant by dramatic multiplication (pp.17–18). Within this article they linked concepts presented by Eco with the concept of dramatic multiplication. From the perspective of the communication sciences, Eco analyses art work based on semiotic models (originally created by Peirce). Eco was mainly interested in the communication structure of art works and the active participation of the public. In 1989 Kesselman and Pavlovsky published (in Argentina) a book entitled 'The dramatic multiplication', which was translated into Portuguese in 1991; the book follows the main theme of 'multiplication rather than reduction'. The authors place the dramatic multiplication at the opposite pole with interpretative reduction, addressing the concept of psychotherapy as something that valorizes the aesthetic joy within the art of curing. They also tried to link the ideas of Gilles Deleuze and Felix Guattari[2] with clinical psychotherapy (Kesselman and Pavlovsky 1989, p.38). More recent modifications on the concept can be found in the Argentinean journal *Lo Grupal*.

Over the years, from being seen as a simple dramatic technique, the concept of dramatic multiplication has grown into a new way of thinking about the group. However, it was never actually seen just as a simple dramatic technique by its creators; they defined it as a sequential group work, conceiving the group as a 'machine that produces meaning' (Kesselman and Pavlovsky 1989, pp.18–38).

'Machine' is a term introduced by schizo-analysis in opposition to human subjectivity. According to Deleuze and Guattari, the machine-like unconscious enfolds various social and material fluxes of signs. The machine is defined as a system of cuts and fluxes. It cuts the flux of energy in order to transform it into a different energy flux (for example a flux of movements, or any other kind of energy). The machine cuts a flux that was continuous, but which originated in a previous cut, and so on. This cut doesn't oppose the flux, but it conditions a new flux. These ideas can be related to the fourth dimension of psychodrama, that is, the associative flow (flux) of scenes. A scene is a cut in the already established flow, and is the foundation for a new flow of scenes. In this respect, machines are machines of other machines, products of other products; machines that cut the associative flux and produce associative flux, and so on. Machines are always agents for other machines. Moreover, every machine (scene) contains one or more codes. The connection or linking of scenes (machines) is the connection of codes (the sociometric network of each scene). The group as a machine producing meaning is not a metaphor, but it literally cuts and produces associative fluxes.

Dramatic multiplication, as a conceptual instrument was developed based on various experiences that have in common the following characteristics:

1. Shared therapeutic work (i.e. co-direction).
2. Self-managed work groups (i.e. the facilitator emerges from the group, developing a space of mutual supervision and multiplication).
3. Group facilitation training with the focus on the conflicts of the facilitator or the co-ordinating team (i.e. scenes that are feared by group facilitators).

These group situations constitute the *ingredients* of the concept of dramatic multiplication.

The theoretical background of the authors can help us understand further details regarding the ingredients of the concept (Kesselman and Pavlovsky 1989, p.109). Kesselman works with the perspective of the operative group of Pichon-Riviere; the analytic psychodrama of Pavlovsky and Frydlewsky; the group analysis of Hanne, Juan Campos and Malcolm Pines; and the corporal drama and corporal dynamics of Suzana de Kesselman (1987, pp.75–80). Pavlovsky's work is based on ideas of Freud, Bion, Ezriel, Slavson, Foulkes, Levobici, Anzieu, Kaes, Langer-Grinberg-Rodrigue; he further expanded these ideas with his own theatrical experiences as an actor and playwright, as well as his training with Zerka and J.L. Moreno (in Beacon 1963). Both authors were strongly influenced by the Argentinean psychoanalytic school, the social psychoanalysis of Pichon-Riviere, and the group psychoanalytic therapy schools. As it was usual for most Argentinean authors, psychodrama came later in their professional development.

What is dramatic multiplication?

In order to call a dramatic experience dramatic multiplication, it needs to follow a certain sequence:

1. In the first step a protagonist gives an account of a personal experience.
2. The second step consists in the dramatization and exploration of the protagonist's scene.

3. The third step consists of dramatic plays created by the group in a state of spontaneity/creativity inspired by the initial scene, and of improvisations that are based on the resonances of each group member with the initial scene.

It is important that the starting scene is chosen by the group based on a sociometric choice. This gives the possibility of the group spontaneously and creatively taking part in the process of group creation. After having worked with the scene brought by the protagonist, the objective of the work shifts to the group, trying to enable their involvement in the scene. In other words, the group takes over the scene from the original protagonist and considers it their own; based on their resonances and consonances with the original scene, the group will continue dramatically to play and improvise with the scene.

In the foreword I wrote for the Brazilian edition of the book 'Dramatic multiplication' (Kesselman and Pavlovsky 1989, p.10), I mentioned that I see dramatic multiplication as 'in act Morenian sharing' (sharing through action). However, I think that some further distinctions are necessary to be made to this statement. *Sharing* in its more common sense means to share with the protagonist feelings and emotions experienced in the here-and-now of the dramatization, or to share moments remembered from our own life (a historical reference). To resonate, on the other hand, means to create without the necessity of referring to a remembered scene of the past. *Consonance* (and to consort) – being the dramatization of a scene from our own personal history – is more close to the act of sharing.

Dramatic multiplication points towards a group-oriented conception of normal and pathological human behaviour. The way to touch upon and unveil the intimate and the painful (wounds) of the other is not to question him/her, but to project ourselves, to consort and resound with the other and in the others. These resonances and consonances 'are like the pieces of a jigsaw puzzle, they complement our own intimacy and vice-versa' (Kesselman and Pavlovsky 1989, p.92). Kesselman relates this idea to that of Foulkes' trans-individuality and transpersonal resonance, where the intimacies of the other reflect and reveal our own intimacies.

The core of the curing process is the accomplishment of spontaneous/creative play among the group members and the therapist. Pavlovsky agrees with Winnicott in stating that psychotherapy is related to the possibility and the accomplishment of play between the therapist and the patients. The aim is to play or to recover the ability to play. Without creation and play there is no cure. Spontaneous, creative and mutual play between patients and therapist enables the repetition of the behaviours that paralyse creation to be stopped. Pavlovsky's concept of the creative matrix, Winnicott's concept of the transitional zone and Moreno's concept of the spontaneous state, all express this idea. Developing or recovering the spontaneity/creativity is the main focus of psychodramatic work. Dramatic multiplication also follows this intention.

The sense of cure is a result of the transition from the uncanny (*unheimliche*), to the pathetic and the playful. 'Uncanny' is a concept taken from Freud (1919, p.273) and Pichon-Riviere (1971), referring to something that is in us, but without us being aware of it (hence the 'strangely familiar' feeling when seeing this something in others). 'Pathetic' refers to the perception of being tied down and not being able to get out of the situation (noticing that something is wrong inside us, but feeling inadequate, or not even wanting to change it). 'Playful' refers to the ability for spontaneity and creativity; the ability to transform the uncanny and the pathetic into aesthetic pleasure, into something marvellous, exorcising the uncanny and the pathetic (Pavlovsky 1980, p.67).

In the 'as if' of the dramatic context, a playful and dreamlike space is concretized, developing spontaneity/creativity; this is a space between the real and imaginary, between the external and internal world. It is a poetic space, where the creator is completely absorbed by the image that was created, giving himself to the sense of surprise and unusual of the first moments, noticing the uncanny. Little by little, by overcoming the surprise and moving from pure fiction to the recognition of the scenes as representative of the facts from his own life, a sense of pleasure develops in creating and representing a certain aesthetic creation.

Dramatic multiplication therefore, is a device of group creation, an agent for a state of group spontaneity/creativity. Stimulated by the original scene, the group members connect it (in a dramatic form) with a feeling, an image or an idea; there is also excitement in the dramatization of multiplied scenes. Since the work is done in the group, the state of group spontaneity has the potential of breaking away from the narcissistic monocular perspective of the individual; this narcissistic view is based in the founding myth of the I, in the matrix of identity of the individual. Sharing the state of spontaneity/creativity and experiencing the state of others is a potential means for the breach from this narcissism (Pavlovsky 1980, p.65).

The spontaneous/creative state has a central position both in Moreno's work and the dramatic multiplication. A great part of Pavlovsky's writings regarding dramatic multiplication refers to this spontaneous state, the process that unchains this state and its therapeutic effects. Based on his own experiences as an actor and playwright, he formulated the concept of the matrix of the creative process, in the therapeutic sense of aesthetic creation and the different climates that accompany this process.

Pavlovsky joined the philosophers of deconstruction, the critics of the more orthodox psychoanalysis and structuralism (Deleuze and Guattari), because psychoanalysis failed to reach this dimension of the curing effect of creativity, and because psychoanalysis made an obscene gesture of violence and sterilization when interpreting creation. The state of spontaneity shouldn't be interpreted oedipally, but is something that should be reached and enabled to flow, allowing sense and meaning to arise (Kesselman and Pavlovsky 1989, p.57).

Applications of the technique

Originally, Pavlovsky and Kesselman worked with experimental groups, with a predominant focus on the dramatic multiplication. These authors also applied dramatic multiplication in groups of didactic analysis with the objective of training (Kesselman and Pavlovsky 1980). Most commonly we would find references regarding the use of dramatic multiplication in experimental groups designated for the research of this technique, however, some authors used it in different settings as well.

Smolovich (1985) for example, describes an experimental group of 'psy' professionals (psychologists, psychiatrists, psychotherapists) where dramatic multiplication was used. Approaching dramatic multiplication from a psychoanalytic perspective, he introduced certain variations to the technique, suggesting its application within training groups, therapeutic self-development groups and institutional groups. Susana Kesselman (Kesselman and Kesselman 1987), working with corporal-drama, used dramatic multiplication in psychotherapy and training groups.

Personally, I tend to use dramatic multiplication both in ongoing groups and in one-off acts, not as much as a form of research, but applying the technique to the situations presented by these groups. I use dramatic multiplication in therapy groups, in psychodrama training or supervision groups, as well as groups of group facilitators and various institutional interventions. In contrast with the creators of the technique (who applied it from a psychoanalytic perspective), I use dramatic multiplication from a psychodramatic perspective. I follow the different structural phases of psychodrama: warm-up, dramatization and sharing. The dramatic multiplication does not substitute the sharing, but prepares it and allows it to happen.

Regarding the clinical indications of dramatic multiplication, my position is the following: I do not consider dramatic multiplication (as a sequential technique) as the only group psychotherapy procedure; I believe that in order to achieve a more complete psychotherapeutic approach, other procedures also need to be applied (for example, focus on the protagonist). A particular case of sociodrama where the technique of dramatic multiplication is worth being used is family psychotherapy. In fact, in the Morenian literature, the 'psychodrama of Adolf Hitler' (Moreno 1959) can be considered as the first ever dramatic multiplication. In the next section, I will look at this case in more detail.

'The psychodrama of Adolf Hitler': a psychodrama paradigm and its connection with dramatic multiplication

After having formulated the foundations of sociometry and having clearly delineated psychodrama as a group psychotherapy method, Moreno (1959) presented his book *Psychodrama Vol. 2 – Foundations of Psychotherapy*, a summarized and well-articulated synthesis of his work. In Chapter 5 of this book Moreno describes the case of Karl (a 40-years-old patient) whom he treated in New York at the beginning of the Second World War. Karl believed himself to be Hitler, and so the case is referred to in the psychodrama literature as the 'psychodrama of Adolf Hitler'.

The structure of the treatment basically consisted in the building of a group device in order to provide the following two working axes:

1. To accept the patient's delusion, that is, within his direct and corresponding interactions with the auxiliary egos (representing characters of his delusion within the dramatic context, for example, Goering and Goebbels) to treat him as if he was Adolf Hitler. Moreno considered that this was the turning point of the treatment:

    > in the case of our pseudo-Hitler, who was non-cooperative to an extreme, it was possible to warm him up to a level of communication when an auxiliary ego portrayed the role of Goering in an episode relevant to his [patient] psychotic world. Once he had established rapport with the auxiliary therapist on

the psychodramatic stage, he was later able to develop a relationship with the private person behind Goering, just a plain therapeutic nurse, with whom he began to communicate spontaneously on a realistic level. (Moreno 1959, p.198)

This axis presents a lot of similarities with strategies that later on were adopted by the anti-psychiatry movement.

2. To create a group device – in this case the psychiatry residents and later on also Karl's wife – that takes part intensely in the sessions, sharing and dramatizing issues related to the rise of the real Hitler. At times, even the group was wondering whether Karl, the patient, was not the real Hitler and the other in Germany his double. The group often took the central working space, transforming it into a sociodrama of that era. They mixed episodes originated in Karl's dreams and delusion with the reality of the historical context experienced in the here-and-now of the group. In Moreno's words: 'A magnificent panorama of the world of our time emerged in bold relief, as if caught in the miniature mirror of this group.' (Moreno 1959, p.199) This second working axis is very close to the concept of dramatic multiplication.

Within this second working axis of the psychodrama of Adolf Hitler, the following characters appear: familial figures of Hitler's life reflected in their relationship to the corresponding figures in the life of each member of the group (these scenes represented Hitler in a more human and conflicted light); Stalin, Mussolini, Roosevelt, Churchill and other political leaders of that historical period; an unknown soldier; the victims of the concentration camps; refugees; a black student from Harlem, identifying himself with Asiatic and African rebels; characters representing nuances of love and hatred, prejudice and tolerance. These characters appear with such intensity that they put Karl's actual, private drama into the shade. In Moreno's words: 'The more Karl himself participated in it [the drama], the more he learnt to see his own private paranoiac world in the perspective of the larger one which he had unconsciously provoked' (Moreno 1959, p.200). Later on Moreno adds: 'The psychodrama of Adolf Hitler turned into the psycho-sociodrama of our entire culture – a mirror of the Twentieth Century' (Moreno 1959, p.200).

What also caught my attention in the psychodrama of Adolf Hitler is the difference between the resources (characteristic of that time) for the treatment of psychotics and Moreno's working framework, which anticipates many of the later approaches. At the time, Freud had already published all his major works, but psychoanalysis had come to a dead end with respect to the treatment of psychosis. Moreno (1934) had already written *Who Shall Survive?* (the foundations of sociometry), but psychiatric treatment was dominated by electro-shock therapy. It was only from the 1950s onwards that they started to systematize group and communitarian family treatment.

The group device applied by Moreno has many similarities with dramatic multiplication. In sequential terms, the work starts with scenes of Karl as protagonist; these are followed by scenes produced by the group based on their resonances with the protagonist and with the historic facts of the time. This group device leads to a spontaneous/creative state (involving both the group and the protagonist). In the language of dramatic multiplication we can say that the monocular vision of the various individual scenes was transformed into the molecular vision of shared group scenes. There is such a great degree of mixing psychodrama and sociodrama that at times we don't know if the multiplications were done by the students or Karl himself.

Moreno made it clear that his intention was to create a device capable of providing structure for the feelings, thoughts, as well as internal and external sensations that arose in a spontaneous and creative manner from reality or imagination. He wanted to create a device that allows the linking of the psychological and social perspective, the linking of dreams and delusion with historical facts, a device that can humanize Hitler, make the audience cry and identify with Karl and the real Hitler, a device that makes it possible to work with all these internalized characters. What happened to Karl or Hitler could happen to anyone else in the group.

In my view, the case of Adolf Hitler represents a psycho-sociodramatic model of family and community therapy, that can be applied for psychotics and other pathologies that would need a familial or community approach. Beyond this specific way of application, it also constitutes a group paradigm for psychodrama in general.

Moreno's chapter on the psychodrama of Adolf Hitler consists of four sub-sections: introduction, technology, psychodramatic production and the group. He starts the 'Introduction' with the following statement: 'psychodrama explores the truth by means of dramatic methods' (Moreno 1959, p.191). But what kind of truth does he mean by this? As the chapter develops it becomes clear that by truth Moreno sometimes means the historical truth of Karl's life, or the truth of the historical moment; other times he means the truth of the moment of the spontaneous creation and the flux that connects reality and fantasy. Still, in the Introduction, Moreno makes a statement of principles regarding psychodrama; these principles can be ordered in the following way:

1. To create a device that represents society in miniature.
2. To allow catharsis of integration and not just analysis and verbal interview.
3. To allow the structuring of internal and external events.
4. To allow to go beyond the individual and collective ideologies, and that besides the symbolic to reach the realm that structures abreactions, feelings and thoughts into embodiment and concrete characters.

What can we say about this statement of principles? First of all, (1) the idea of the group as a miniature society stresses the necessity to elaborate concepts that connect the specificity of intra-group happenings with the cultural and social phenomenon. Secondly, (2) by stressing the importance of the catharsis of integration, Moreno removes the emphasis from the purely verbal language, and focuses on an inter-semiotic code of expression and understanding. Thirdly, (3) Moreno suggests the creation of a device that connects the internal with the external (connects the intra-psychic with the inter-psychic, as well as the intra-groupal with the inter-groupal). Fourthly, (4) in this perspective, logical (symbolic) elaboration is not based on individual or group ideologies, but on the flow of happenings that occur in the here-and-now of the group members (these group members are in a state of spontaneity).

In the sub-section entitled 'Technology', Moreno emphasizes psychodrama as a device that connects reality with fantasy, the protagonist with the group, and the different codes of expression.

In the sub-section on 'Psycodramatic production', he describes the working axis based on the protagonist's production; the protagonist having complete autonomy. On the one hand, Moreno proposes corrective scenes involving the protagonist's real mother, on the other hand scenes of self-realization of the (protagonist's) desire as well as multiplications with the participation of the audience. Within this mixture of strategies, Moreno prefers the dramatic production of the protagonist, accepting his delusion and working with the delusion as a starting point. Moreno describes moments of creative confusion when the group seemed to see the real Hitler in Karl, or in other words, the group expropriated Karl's delusion not just simply as a strategy but as the truth. There were also other moments when Karl managed to get out of the uncanny and face and confront the pathetic aspects of his situation (the moment when he shaved off his moustache – cutting his moustache in reality and not in the 'as if'). In that moment, the group managed to create in the here-and-now something more intense and powerful than the delusional world of Karl, than the sociodrama of the period or than any logical interpretation. According to Moreno this moment was of 'unique value for the progress of the therapy…a direct and real contact between the people in a state of spontaneity, not in the context of the as if, but in the context of the group'. Shaving off the moustache concentrates in a single moment Karl's recognition of his pathetic situation; it allowed him to experiment with an original and *sui generic* fact, with a very intense dramatic quality. Out of the spontaneity/creativity of the act, he created new meaning.

In the sub-section referring to the 'Group', Moreno emphasizes the importance of the intense involvement and participation of the audience, already from the second session (a sociodrama when Hitler sat in the audience as a member of the group). The device proposed by Moreno allowed a mixture of two production focuses: focus on Karl (the protagonist) and focus on the audience (consisting of residents). From Karl's point of view, this was an inside-out and outside-in axis of production. Karl's delusion was transformed into a form of group interaction, and the interaction of the group was transformed into a form of Karl's delusion. 'Many episodes resulting from the interactions were acted out on the stage, mixing the events in Hitler's dream with the actualities of the group' (Moreno 1959, p.199)

In his Foreword to the Brazilian edition (1983) of Moreno's *Foundations of Psychotherapy* Naffah Neto considers the case of Adolf Hitler as doubly innovative: Moreno's approach is a psychotherapeutic method preceding and being a precursor to the anti-psychiatry model; the second innovation is the linking of intra-psychic phenomenon with inter-subjective (inter-personal) and historical contradictions, thus pointing out essential and intrinsic relationships between subjectivity and history. One could say that Moreno didn't just anticipate anti-psychiatry, but also dramatic multiplication.

However, we also need to stress that there are some significant differences between dramatic multiplication and Moreno's work. The most important is the confusion resulting from taking the accounts of Karl's story as true facts that happened. This confusion resulted in corrective dramatizations of some traumas that were taken as real (true). However, if we consider the patient's accounts to be myths (the historical truth as experienced by him), we open the door for the forming of judgements regarding the accounts of the patient, or in other words, the account is placed in between a supposedly true fact and the actual (real) fact. What intervenes between the sense of happening (it doesn't matter if it is a real happening or not; what is important is that it is sensed as real) and the narration, is the language. Moreno didn't formulate a clear view regarding this concept of the language.

The concept of language (as we understand it today) was formulated at the beginning of the twentieth century, based on three different sources: the soviet school, Saussure's linguistics and Pierce's semiotics. It was only after the Second World War, with the development of mass society (and so mass sociology), that these concepts started to grow within the human sciences. Inspired by Saussure, it was Lacan who introduced them into the 'psy' (psychological) sciences. Presently there are many other schools that work with concepts related to language, but in a different way from Lacan; since it was inspired by Pierce through Umberto Eco, dramatic multiplication is one of them.

Language is 'the totality of signs that serve as means of communication between individuals and can be received by the different sensory organs; this results in a distinction between visual language, auditive language, a tactile language, etc., or even more complex languages that consist of a concomitant combination of these elements' (Almeida 1982). Language is an organization or systematization of stimuli carried out by man. Language is the foundation of all communication; it is the foundation of culture, the matrix of human behaviour and thinking. 'all systems and forms of language tend to behave as living systems, or in other words, they reproduce, re-adapt, transform and regenerate as living things' (Almeida 1982). It is the language that determines the connection between events without sense and meaning, that is, language gives meaning. It intervenes between the pure experience (of the event) and its narration.

Dramatic multiplication resumes the working model of the psychodrama of Adolf Hitler and further enriches it with different concepts originating in semiotics and schizo-analysis. In the following I will list some of the contributions of this technique that I consider most significant:

1. It enriches our understanding of the spontaneous/creative states through the concepts of the molar and molecular vision, the concept of encounter based on multiplicative resonance, and the

understanding of the aesthetic message as ambiguous and auto-reflexive.

2. In the light of the concept of schizo-analytic unconscious, it allows us to redefine the concept of co-unconscious.
3. It enables us to analyse psychodramatic production in terms of the linguistic axes of the metaphor and metonymy (both basic techniques in psychodrama).
4. It approaches the sense of cure through the concepts of the uncanny, pathetic and playful (based on the conceptualization of Freud and Pichon-Riviere).
5. It offers a potentially new way of treating ego-sintonic pathologies as well as family or community groups.

Conclusions

I would like to stress that since it was formulated (in 1987), the concept of dramatic multiplication has further developed. Even though it originated in the training experiences with group facilitators and psychodramatists, it has been applied in various other group processes. It is a way of conceiving the group as a machine producing meaning, as well as a sequential group work. Conceptually, dramatic multiplication is at the intersection of psychodrama with theatre, psychoanalysis, semiotics and schizo-analysis. The therapeutic aspect of this instrument is connected to:

1. its capacity to break away from monocular narcissism
2. the aesthetic pleasure of collective group creation
3. the possibility of touching the intimate of the other through our own resonances
4. its possibility of revealing the uncanny and mobilize the pathetic, arriving at the playful.

Notes

1 This chapter is based on the following two articles by Pedro Mascarenhas: 'Multiplicação dramática'. *Revista Brasileira de Psicodrama* 4, 1, 1996, pp.13–21; and 'O Psicodrama de Adolf Hitler: Um paradigma do psicodrama e a sua relação com a multiplicação dramática'. *Revista Brasileira de Psicodrama* 5, 1, 1997, pp.43–50.
2 Based on their studies of psychosis, Deleuze and Guattari developed a critical theory of psychoanalysis, which they called 'schizo-analysis'.

13

I hate you...please don't leave me!
The borderline client and psychodrama[1]

Rosa Cukier and Sonia Marmelsztejn

Perhaps some therapists have already had the experience of working with clients who become furious during sessions, complaining about the therapist's professional ability, about something that was said or even the way it was done. We therapists become very unsure of ourselves at these moments. We do not know how to act, on the one hand trying to find out what we did wrong, and on the other being absolutely sure that it was more the client's performance making us angry and sometimes even afraid of him.

As therapists, we know that it is not easy to admit that we may feel anger and fear towards our clients. However, in the specific case of borderline clients, these are the exact feelings that they commonly produce in the people who are the most intimate and dear to them. Therefore, it is essential for the therapist to be aware of this and to be able to decode his own emotions without blame or shame, so as not to act in a complementary way and to help these clients understand the psychodynamics involved in the process.

According to Lineham's (1993, p.3) estimation, in the United States 11 per cent of non-committed psychiatric clients, and 19 per cent of committed ones are borderline clients. Among those who are diagnosed with 'personality disorders', 33 per cent of non-committed clients and 63 per cent of committed ones are considered to be borderlines. Therefore, this type of client is frequent enough for us to believe that most therapists have come across at least one case during their practise.

Besides this, these clients are also the ones who most often commit suicide. It is estimated that 70 to 75 per cent of borderline clients have at least one self-destructive episode or act, with approximately 9 per cent of the cases being fatal (Lineham 1993, p.3).

In Brazil, we do not know of any work concerning the prevalence of this pathology within mental disorders. However, considering our own clinics and the experiences of our colleagues, we think that something similar must be taking place. What is intriguing is that besides the great danger of this condition, all available therapies fail without exception, while therapeutic progress is extremely insignificant and slow. These clients normally come to the clinics with a list of therapists whom they have already consulted, having been over-medicated (as doctors often try several psychiatric medicines in an attempt to control the symptoms), while their families seem devastated and with no hope of getting proper help.

The concept of borderline personality

The term 'borderline' was used for the first time by Adolf Stern in 1938 to describe a group of clients who appeared not to be benefiting from classical psychoanalysis, and who did not fit in the 'neurotic' or 'psychotic' categories. In reality, according to his classification they had a type of borderline neurosis. In 1980, the condition was included in the *Diagnostic and Statistical Manual of Mental Disorders* (DSM III) of the American Psychiatric Association.

Clients with borderline personality present certain interpersonal, emotional and behavioural characteristics. In the following I will list some of the most common of these; however, I would also like to point out that different borderline clients will present different combinations of these characteristics, without the necessary presence of all of them.

Interpersonal characteristics

In terms of interpersonal relationships theborderline client thinks in a dichotomous and radical way. His world, similar to that of a child, is full of heroes and villains, and frequently a slip-up or failure by the hero leads to his inevitable condemnation and devaluation. He does not understand grey areas, inconsistencies or ambiguities. Good and evil do not mix: somebody is either totally good or totally evil. He idealizes and gets disappointed all the time, appearing to be in an eternal search for the perfect caregiver, the one who will always be right.

The borderline person lacks a clear perception of the boundaries between himself and the other, this resulting in his unstable sense of self. He usually has a need to impress people in order to keep them around, while his sense of identity and self-esteem are associated with getting (or not getting) this attention. Therefore, he needs continuous proof of this, but deep down he has a feeling of non-authenticity, of falseness. Even when successful, the borderline gets upset, believing that he did not deserve the attention or that people will discover that he is a fraud and he will be humiliated.

This is why borderlines cannot stick to a job; they will keep on getting new ones, hoping that the next one will be different and they will feel better there. They are literally unable to 'find themselves'. This confusion is often further complicated by issues around sexual identity; just as the borderline does not know who he is, he is also unable to decide what he desires.

Similar to the child who is not able to distinguish between the occasional absence of the mother and her death or total disappearance, the borderline experiences occasional loneliness as a sensation of complete and eternal isolation. Since he cannot tolerate loneliness as a result of real or imaginary abandonment, he becomes seriously depressed as he loses the sensation of being alive. His existential motto appears to be: 'If others interact with me, then I exist.'

Emotional characteristics

The borderline client's mood is often unstable and it can vary greatly in only one day or even in the course of a few hours. He is usually not calm and controlled, but often irritable, hyperactive, pessimistic and depressed. His reactions are generally very intense and inappropriate for the situation that produced them.

The borderline client struggles with his intense feelings of anger, which he does not seem to be able to control. His fits of rage are unpredictable and disproportionate to the frustrations that produced them. Domestic scenes of screaming, breaking objects, threatening with knives and hitting/scratching people are typical for these clients. Anger may be triggered by any trivial offence, but in fact it seems to come from some underground arsenal, from the fear of being abandoned or disappointed.

The borderline will direct his anger at those who are closest to him: relatives, therapists or doctors. It aims to test the bonds and commitments in an incessant search to find out how far he can push people. It seems to be an incompetent cry for help, as it ends up pushing away the people whom he needs most. For this reason, many therapists stop the treatment early or limit the number of borderline clients whom they treat.

The absence of a strong sense of identity can culminate in a feeling of existential emptiness. This is so painful that the borderline will resort to impulsive and self-destructive behaviours in order to get rid of this feeling.

Behavioural characteristics

The borderline lacks the ability to postpone gratification: his behaviour is impulsive, based on intense momentary feelings and is potentially damaging to him. Compulsive spending and/or sexual behaviour, substance misuse, or binge eating are quite common among borderline clients, and they do not seem to learn from experience. They have an altered notion of time: 'yesterday' and 'tomorrow' are meaningless; only 'today' seems to exist.

Borderline clients commonly present suicidal or self-harming behavioural patterns. This self-destructive behaviour has a double significance. Firstly, it is a proof of the depression and despair underlying this condition: to feel physical pain is, in extreme cases, the only way of feeling alive and/or a very efficient way of distracting oneself from greater suffering. Secondly, the para-suicidal behaviour[3] indicates a need of these clients to manipulate the people who take care of them in order to get more attention or love. In general, they do not want to die but only to communicate their suffering in a convincing way. Paradoxically, because of being insistent and repetitive they end up driving people away, which makes them needier, more desperate and results in a greater desire to hurt themselves.

Many clients report feeling calm and relieved after such 'accidents'; some scientists believe that this phenomenon can be attributed to the release of endorphins, a kind of self-treatment of the organism when in pain. However, both the self-destructive behaviour and the sense of well-being resulting from it are phenomena that are not easy to explain and understand. In psychotherapy, it is this symptom that causes therapists their greatest problems: if a great amount of attention is paid to these self-destructive behaviours, there is a risk of reinforcing them; on the other hand, if they are ignored, the client can insist and go on in a progression of attempts to cause a stronger impact, which can result in actual suicide.

When not associated with psychosis, self-mutilation is a trademark of the borderline disorder. There are many different ways for a person to inflict harm on himself: he can cut himself, smoke or eat in excess, neglect his body, drive recklessly, etc.

Further to the above described interpersonal, emotional and behavioural characteristics, under highly stressful circumstances, the borderline may show symptoms of temporary dissociation, confused and delusional thinking and paranoid interpretation of the facts. Generally, he places himself in the victim role of an unjust situation.

Etiology

Regarding the etiology of the borderline disorder, the following three causes can be taken into consideration: inadequate emotional development, constitutional factors and sociocultural factors.

Inadequate emotional development

The clinical history of borderline clients frequently proves that they come from very disturbed families, characterized by a high occurrence of family fights and separations. Generally speaking, during their childhood these clients suffered a wide range of abuse, such as physical, sexual and emotional abuse. The self-destructive behaviour of borderline clients can be seen as an unconscious way of perpetuating the abuse of the parents.

According to the specialized literature (Mahler 1977; Erikson 1968), the roots of this pathology can generally be traced back to the age of 18 to 30 months, that is, the period following shortly after the child has acquired the ability to walk. Within this period parents tend to oscillate between controlling the child in order to help him avoid hurting himself (since he just recently started to walk), and becoming slightly absent – freeing themselves too early from the child who now prefers to explore the world instead of passively sitting on his parents' lap.

Constitutional factors

In the literature there are only certain suggestions regarding the presence of constitutional or hereditary factors in the etiology of the borderline disorder. We know for example, that siblings brought up within the same family have different reactions to conflicts and only some of them develop borderline disorder. This shows that something specific is needed in order to create a certain type of disorder and not another, however, until now it has not been possible to determine whether this indicates a biological or psychological inheritance of the disorder.

Socio-cultural factors

Some authors have correctly pointed out that at the present time there are certain socio-cultural factors that contribute to the high occurrence of both narcissistic and borderline disorders. The lack of a nuclear family structure, consisting of both a mother and a father who spend time taking care of their children, is one of the most often mentioned points within the analysis of these socio-cultural factors.

The changes that occurred in the role of women over the last 30 years have radically altered the domestic routine. Children also go to school early or are looked after by others (because old people are treated with disregard); all these changes contribute to a loss of the sense of pertinence, history and family closeness, as well as the loss of consistent social roles.

We live in a '*borderland*' where we stimulate assertiveness (which in its extreme forms can reach aggression), individualism (favouring loneliness and alienation) and self-preservation ('everybody for himself, God for all'). Our society lacks consistency and reliability and is extremely alienating, thus favouring the appearance of a range of pathological behaviours, such as drug addiction, eating disorders, criminal behaviour, etc. It is a well-known fact that numerous physical illnesses (for example stress and stress related disorders, such as heart attacks, hypertension, etc.) are closely related to our lifestyle. Why couldn't this also be true in the case of mental illness? Mental illness is perhaps the psychological price we pay for the modern life we live.

Psychodynamics – how does the borderline client function?

Imagine a person who, due to some congenital mistake, is born without skin: he feels agony at the slightest touch or movement. The borderline is similar to this, only he is lacking 'emotional skin'.

An environment that offers little validation is one which does not teach the child how to deal adequately with his emotions. This learning process (mainly non-verbal) does not simply consist in the recognition and knowing of the different emotions, but it also presupposes the learning of how to externalize or contain them, how to deal with frustrations, and above all, to believe in one's own emotional responses as valid forms of interpreting the facts (basic self-confidence).

The dysfunctional families of borderline clients deal inconsistently with emotions, teaching their children to focus their energy in accomplishing something 'big' in order to be noticed and valued by their parents.

As a consequence, the borderline adult will try at all costs to stay close to a caregiver. He has a passive attitude towards things he should do, but he is extremely active in finding someone who will do them for him. This can be accomplished in various ways: for example, by being chronically ill, either psychologically, or physically; by presenting oneself as a very naive person without any malice, only to later develop a manipulative relationship; by creating a lot of trouble in these relationships and by being the eternal victim, never being treated justly and continuously fighting for his rights, etc.

People living close to the borderline (such as family members and therapists) have a feeling of 'walking on eggshells', since he is never satisfied and creates situations that do not seem to have a way out. He always has to have something to complain about, perhaps to keep someone close, trying to satisfy him.

Furthermore, as he comes from an environment that neglected his basic childhood needs for dependence (Erikson 1968), the borderline remains fixated on the search for a good caregiver, the search for the 'perfect' carer. He idealizes and becomes disappointed very easily, becoming furious when noticing the imperfections of the other. He is like a child who imagines that his mother knows and can do everything, and cannot accept that this may not be true.

As an adult, the borderline ends up reproducing the devaluating characteristics of his childhood environment: he considers his own emotional experiences as worthless, searching for other (alternative) interpretations of reality. He is unable to solve routine problems and has great difficulties regarding 'how to live'.

Being a 'prisoner' of his own emotions, a small thing may provoke a strong reaction (such as fits of rage and violence) in the borderline, confusing and frightening himself and those around him. He creates 'tragic' situations and complains with vehement rage, blaming others for the situation into which he has got; the greater his fit of rage, the more the borderline convinces himself and tries to convince others that they are the ones responsible for his feelings. His emotional responses are also long-lasting, and it takes quite some time for the borderline to return to a more adequate emotional level. This also results in the fact that he is highly sensitive to the next emotional stimulus.

With his emotional development stuck in its early phases, the borderline is a child inside an adult's body. As with all children, he is impulsive, he does not know how to wait, cannot cope with frustration, he has difficulties in symbolizing abstract concepts (like time for example), and he always tries to get everything that he wants, at any cost. Because of his difficulty in making decisions and taking responsibility, he tends to be professionally more successful in subordinate positions, preferring well structured jobs that do not demand these abilities.

Psychotherapy with borderline clients

There are two fundamental difficulties in the therapeutic treatment of borderline clients. The first is what we could call the collision of objectives; this means that the usual aims of a therapy process (understanding one's own problems, 'healing oneself', undertaking constructive changes in one's life, etc.) do not coincide with this client's main aims. To start with, the borderline client does not want to heal himself; to some extent, he is even proud of his symptoms, as they are witnesses to the atrocities that he has gone through in life. What he is looking for, within a therapeutic relationship, is exactly this witness function: someone who can see and disagree with the injustice committed against him. He also wants the therapist to compensate him for everything that he has gone through; he wants the therapist to satisfy his (the client's) immediate needs, and to take care of him and comfort him. In order to feel important, he wants the therapist to provide an intense and special relationship. This can seriously complicate the therapist's job. What all this implicitly communicates is: 'I cannot get better unless you, the therapist, demonstrate that you personally care about me.'

Case example: M

M, a 16-year's-old client, is thinking about studying psychology and is not happy with her own appearance; this is all that brought her to therapy. In the initial interview, her parents complained about her attempts to manipulate everyone in the family to get what she wants.

From the beginning, she presented herself as an extremely insecure and distressed person, anxious to please. Right away she started to idealize the therapist, not missing any opportunity to praise her (the therapist) and recommend her to her (the client's) best friends.

To investigate the function of this exaggerated idealization, an internal psychodrama was proposed (since the client refused normal dramatization). After the warm-up the therapist suggested focusing on the therapeutic relationship by using role reversals, so that the client could experience both sides of this relationship.

In the role of herself, M stated that she was fascinated by the therapist and wanted to get her affection in a 'special way', because this therapist (unlike the previous one) seemed to be competent and capable of understanding her. In the role of the therapist, the client presented herself as unreachable, a person who had everything and appreciated very much the 'presents' (recommendations) offered by her client, however, she was not ready to allow her client enter the so-called 'special place'.

In the next step of this internal psychodrama, the therapist asked the client to distance herself from this relationship and observe it; she also asked whether the client had other relationships where she had felt the same way: liking someone so much that he/she seemed unreachable and that no matter how much she tried to please, she could not obtain what she most wanted from this person.

The client recalled a scene from her childhood (she was around four or five years old) in which, being out for a walk with her real father, she did everything to seem unpleasant and to deny his importance: she wanted to make it clear that she loved her stepfather more (the stepfather had just recently married her mother and now assumed the position of full-time father). M felt very grateful to her stepfather and could not stand the idea of displeasing him. Praising him in front of her real father was a way of paying him homage and at the same time getting revenge for her father's abandonment.

Reviewing this scene helped the client notice her attempts throughout her life of feeling 'special'. These attempts failed systematically without exception: she had not been special to her father, who rarely visited her; she was not special to her mother, who had many other priorities; and she did not even remain special to her stepfather after the birth of his new children with the client's mother. Her performance in the therapy was just one more of these attempts to reach this 'special' place.

The second difficulty in the therapy of borderline clients is the style of the relationship they try to establish with the therapist: while they try to get their needs met, they do not believe that this can happen. Considering that many of these clients have suffered various forms of child abuse from their caregivers, it is easy to imagine how any relationship implying personal care will soon be impregnated with distrust from their past. Therefore, establishing a firm therapeutic relationship and a sense of being understood and accepted is the first necessary step for the borderline client to be able to engage in the painful attempt of looking at his difficulties and trying to change his life. The borderline client does not know how it feels to be accepted and understood, and so he will keep checking it repeatedly. He will move forward and then retreat and, in order to maintain the balance, the therapist will also need to do the same: a too sudden advance or retreat on the therapist's part may jeopardize the already achieved work. The client will test constantly how important he is for the therapist and at the slightest sign that could be interpreted as rejection he may attack, sabotage, or interrupt the therapy.

Case example: I

I, a 34-year-old client, has a long history of unsuccessful therapies; she is deeply depressed, cries a lot, and feels hopeless. From the beginning she was very critical of everything that the therapist said and the way she did things; in other words, she always disagreed with the therapist, making her feel cornered, having to take a lot of care not to hurt the client.

None of the therapist's attempts to clarify these misunderstandings were successful, because the client became confrontational, opposing everything. The therapist always had the feeling that they would need a judge to decide which one of them was right.

In one of the sessions, while the therapist was trying to filter the client's complaints through what was verbally said, she started to pay more attention to how much the client suffered during the episodes when she was crying, feeling distressed and feeling treated unjustly. She decided to make an apology by telling the client the following:

'Some things that I say or do, seem to touch on an old wound of yours, even if this is not my intention. I would like to apologize to you for this, because it is not my intention to cause you any pain or harm. I believe that with patience we may discover together where this very sensitive point of yours is. For now, I would like you to accept my apology, even though I don't know what I did to hurt you.'

The client responded with complete bewilderment to this comment and started to cry saying that the therapist was not to blame; it was her (the client) who always started arguments in all of her relationships, creating a confrontational atmosphere in her life. Then the therapist invited her to create a character that would represent this feeling of injustice always attacking her, and she produced a Medieval Crusader, a defender of the cause of the Holy Catholic Church.

The client continued therapy for four years, attending both individual and group sessions; she never abandoned the image of this Crusader that became a reference for her confrontational states and helped her investigate several situations of domestic violence which she had suffered in childhood. During these four years she mentioned several times 'the day when the therapist apologized to her', stressing repeatedly that it was the most important moment of her therapy, without which she could have not continued.

Besides these two fundamental difficulties there are many others that a therapist may come across when working with borderline clients: at times, while talking about something simple and not very important, the client may rapidly escalate to extremely controversial and confrontational themes. At other times they may do the opposite, trying to please the therapist, assuming his point of view and ways of thinking; the therapist must be careful to prevent this from happening. Many borderline clients act seductively with the therapist; this is probably a demonstration of the way they used to get attention and kindness in the past. Similar to guerrilla warfare, the therapist is often taken by surprise: the client's seductive forms of relating may alternate with very aggressive ones.

Lineham (1993) and Kroll (1993) draw our attention to the importance of validation, support and empathy for the borderline clients; this is necessary because their childhood experiences invalidated their right to exist, the possibility of their developing individuality, and their trust in their own ability to perceive and judge reality.

Validation, affirmation, giving permission, and reward are therapeutic actions that may be necessary, even if causing a slight confusion in the therapy process. Validation and affirmation are actions that aim at helping the client develop an intrinsic sense of personal value, through a therapeutic relationship of acceptance which tries to highlight the client's positive qualities (as few as they are). This is not always an easy task, because clients present a huge range of inadequate behaviours, and the therapist needs to be careful not to artificially reinforce these, because they wouldn't contribute to the therapy. The fact that the client has survived under such extreme circumstances and is seeking therapy is already praiseworthy in itself; the client needs a lot of courage to embark on such a journey. Real affirmation and restraint are also a result of the therapist's respect for the client, establishing boundaries that the therapist himself also respects such as time, space and phone calls.

Case example: P

P, a 30-year-old client, gets home wanting attention from his wife, who is busy and tired with the couple's two-year-old son. His wife's attitude is immediately interpreted as rejection and P begins attacking her, first verbally and then physically as well. His dissatisfaction and frustration increase rapidly and to such an extent that he cannot contain himself.

Starting from this scene, we eventually arrive at another scene where he is three years old and wants to be held by his mother, who is busy cooking. The mother abruptly pushes him away and he begins angrily to kick her. I ask the client what he, as an adult, would do with the child in this situation. He answers that he would hold him before he starts kicking his mother. I invite him to do this (putting a cushion in the role of the child) and he hugs the cushion and starts crying.

In the sharing, I validated both the pain of the frustrated child as well as the pain of the needy man arriving home; then we discussed the way he dealt with his frustration and the manner of expressing his needs. One of the questions that arose was how to contain a hurt and angry man, to which the client suggested various possibilities including taking a bath, going out for a walk, or writing a letter.

Another form of affirmation (reassurance) is to confirm the client's perception of his own parents and of what they did to him. The therapist is a witness to this abuse, helping the client to cry out his pain and suffering, and to refocus and reorganize his anger. In most cases the client turns his anger against himself, which constitutes one of the reasons for the bizarre self-destructive behaviour characteristic to these cases. However, we also need to be cautious about excessively criticizing the parents because this means criticizing parts of the client himself.

Case example: N

N, is a 17-year-old client, who has been in therapy for two years. For a month she had wanted to tell the therapist about something, but found very difficult to approach the subject. Finally, she managed to tell her 'secret', which happened when she was five and of which she was ashamed: they were at a beach house with a group of children and relatives and she allowed herself to be sexually manipulated by a teenage cousin.

Her mother accidentally discovered what had happened and became furious, criticizing her harshly in front of everybody and telling the story in a very disrespectful way to all the adults who were present. N concluded that she had done something very ugly, that she was bad and wrong, and that she should be ashamed of herself forever.

I suggested a role reversal with the frightened and guilty five-year-old girl, asking what could have helped her better to process this experience. N responded that everything would have been much easier if the mother had supported her and explained what she had done wrong, while keeping the matter only to the two of them. What her mother did in reality, only taught her disrespect, shame and guilt.

I agreed with her statement, witnessed her pain and enabled her to express the anger she had felt towards her mother. The next step was to review the shame and the consequences of that sexual experience. For a child everything seems very serious and definite; for an adult the perception of things becomes more relative. N had held and contained her own internal little girl and gave a new meaning to the consequences of this experience: nothing is completely spoiled for good!

Borderline clients often try to make others pathologically complement them, overstepping the boundaries of therapy. It is always good to remember that a client's greatest desire is to be helped to overcome the difficulties he has lived through, and the therapist's conduct must be based on this.

Case example: N continued

N frequently requested changes in the schedule of the therapy sessions, telling me that some of her routine activities did not allow her to attend a session, and asking for appointment times that were incompatible with my timetable. It was also difficult to finish our sessions on time, because she would always bring up a very important subject right at the end of the sessions. At the beginning, I tried to work around timetables, in order to make the therapy viable.

After almost a year and a half of working together, at the end of a session N refused to leave the therapy room; she had no apparent reason for this, and urged me to remove her by force. After having spent some time discussing the issue with her, I realized that I had to attend to another of my clients. I decided to leave N to stay in the therapy room as long as she 'needed' and see my next client in another therapy room. N stayed for a while and then went away. She arrived at our next session with apologies, saying that she did not know what had provoked her into that attitude during the previous session. While, through the use of role reversal, we investigated what had happened, N realized that she had been observing the client who came after her and felt very jealous because she was more beautiful; she was worried that I 'would certainly find this other client more interesting'.

These associations led back to her relationship with her step-brothers and parents, who 'never chose her' unless she did something out of the ordinary (either in the positive or negative sense). N realized how difficult it was for her to feel valued when she just behaved normally and accepted the boundaries that were set for her.

Permission[4] is a more complex concept, also implying the validation of the client's right of feeling and expressing his own emotions (anger, love, selfishness) and of being respected as a human being. It is normal, for example, for a client not to be able to cut himself free (detach) from people who were abusive to him in the past. Therefore, the client needs to obtain this permission in the therapy.

The vulnerability of the therapist when working with borderline clients

Therapy with a borderline client is a very delicate matter. The borderline client is an eternal unloved child in search of a good caregiver, trying to make the therapist fulfil this role. It is a hard task for the therapist to accept and validate the client's feelings without entering in collusion with him, and without becoming responsible for him. The therapist needs to believe that the client has inside himself all the necessary potential for change. He must also therapeutically encourage the client to recognize and trust his own feelings as being valid ways of interpreting reality, instead of adopting other people's emotions and opinions.

Fulfilling the needs of the borderline client is the most crucial element of the therapy. As we have already mentioned, all actions of the client are aimed to put him in a special and important place in front of the therapist.

After having studied various cases, Kroll (1993) pointed out that there are possible therapeutic and legal complications which can result from the lack of discussion about this particular issue, for example, clients' allegations of sexual abuse or malpractise against therapists, or threats of suicide used for blackmailing the therapist in order to make him do or not to do certain things.

Issues like bodily contact with the client (for example hugs at very tense moments), changing appointments to special days and times, allowing long phone calls at inconvenient times, etc., are the kind of small concessions that the therapist tends to do almost unconsciously, and which can evolve to the point of invalidating the therapeutic setting.

One wonders why even experienced therapists respond in this way to the pleas of the borderline client. This response is probably due to these clients' extreme vulnerability and a certain degree of the therapist's countertransference (of being the all-powerful saviour of the world[5]) that we all have.

Both the excess or failure to fufil the needs of the borderline client can damage or even sabotage his therapy. Similar to all psychotics, the borderline client has the capacity of crossing the professional boundaries, as if needing to feel that the therapist is a real person. Too rigid professional rules do not work very well with these clients, since they feel devalued, unsupported and so become furious.

It is very hard for this kind of client to hear the truth. This 'child inside an adult's body' will do everything to deny that his childhood has finished and that the rules and privileges of the adult world are different. Because of this, support and empathy are fundamental through the whole therapeutic process. Without this support and empathy, the borderline will not listen to the therapist's statements about reality because he feels misunderstood and will argue with the therapist.

There are innumerable difficulties in the therapy process: the borderline client lives in a state of intense suffering, and situations during the therapy process may become so complicated at times that it is difficult to stay focused on the actual cause of this suffering. The therapist may end up feeling as if they are building a house in the middle of a hurricane, which can be very discouraging. Besides this, as the borderline deals badly with all of his emotions (including anger), the therapist may often become subject to aggressive and explosive behaviour. The risk here is that the therapist may 'over-interpret' the anger, failing to notice what is behind the anger – an intense vulnerability.

Finally, I would like to make a warning regarding the danger of what Lineham (1993, p.97) calls 'blaming the victim'. At the beginning of the treatment the therapist sensitizes himself to the client's intense suffering and tries to revert it. However, as he realizes that his efforts seem useless, he may start blaming the client for causing his own misfortune (it is the client who doesn't want to change and resists the therapy). What happens is that the therapist ends up looking at the consequences of the behaviour (the client's suffering and the suffering that he inflicts on the therapist) and will attribute these consequences to the client's internal and deliberate motives. In such a situation it is very easy for the therapist to resign himself to failure, and blame the client for interrupting the treatment, relieving himself of responsibility.

The borderline client in psychodrama psychotherapy

> It seems that there is nothing for which human beings are less prepared and the human brain is less equipped, than for surprise.
> (Moreno 1923, p.47)

Considering the relational character of psychodrama, it is not difficult to see why it might be appropriate for treating borderline clients, in which the client–therapist relationship is fundamental. Beyond the intense therapeutic relationship that offers the chance for the 'live correction' of the ways of relating, psychodrama (thanks to its technical resources) can subtly enter the area of the client's intra-psychic defence, enabling him to relate to the various parts of himself.

It is a dialectic approach, that enters the 'behind the scenes' of psychic life where the relational wounds of the past are stored (creating an arsenal of characterologic defence); and then returns to the here-and-now of a validating and warm relationship which, besides being a witness to the pain of the past, offers a new and reparatory relational model. The borderline client, who is used to defending himself verbally, is surprised by psychodrama. He is not able to control or predict neither the therapist's actions nor his own reactions and associations.

This represents a great advantage for the therapist, who, however, must be careful with timing and the client's sensitivity. Many times the client appears quite warmed-up, bringing up material of an intimate nature as if he were impulsively revealing all of his pain. A too-abrupt approach from the therapist's side however, runs the risk of coming across a not sufficiently elaborated structure on the client's part, who later inevitably will feel harmed. What is often needed is the cooling down of the client, in order to allow him to slowly descend into the depths of his issues and to treat the level of his self-exposure in a responsible way.

Case example: NL

NL is a 50-year-old client who, after two years of individual therapy, just started to attend group therapy sessions; the group members hardly know each other and seem careful and hesitant. NL is the last to introduce herself. She speaks aggressively, saying that she hasn't come to the group to waste her time; she tells the group that as a child she was raped, and that still today she is searching for dangerous experiences, such as having sex with anyone whom she comes across. The group is astonished and nobody says anything; NL becomes angry and provokes an argument.

The therapist intervenes by telling her that what she called a 'waste of time' was a normal way for people to gradually get to know each other, in order to be able to build up relationships of mutual trust, where everyone's intimacy and privacy could be respected. In the rape scene that she talked about, her privacy had not been respected, and the way that she presented herself to the group ended up being a kind of self-rape, where she respected neither herself nor the group.

In the above case, the therapist only pointed out the speed and intensity with which the client wanted to initiate relationships. Other types of overly warmed-up clients need certain technical interventions to help them cool down. Setting up scenes carefully, asking for role reversals with the objects in the scene, and carefully interviewing supporting characters, are all strategies that can be used to cool a client down.

While setting up scenes P would already enter and play the roles and counter-roles involved, speaking angrily and barely giving enough time to build the scene. It seemed as if for her the details of the space were just a waste of time, as if she was pushed by some sense of urgency to finish the job quickly. Once, after she had quickly described her bedroom, the therapist asked her to reverse roles with the door key. She seemed very surprised and then said abruptly that she had never had a key for her door. So the therapist asked her to take on the role of this door without a key. All choked up, she said that the door did not protect her privacy and that during the night her father used to come in through this door, watching her being naked.

Although it is valuable, the use of the double technique can be dangerous with borderline clients. As mentioned earlier, the therapist needs to be careful with the timing of the double, because, if it is not in tune with the client's vulnerability, he may readily deny the double. The best double for an infuriated client is actually the one which points out the sadness, the hurt, and the deception that led to this defensive response. Feelings of humiliation and shame are also often involved.

Doubles pointing out the manipulative character of a client's aggressive behaviour need to be introduced very carefully; these should also be done only after the more fragile aspects of the aggression have been discussed.

Case example: R

R is 30 years old; she has been in individual therapy for two years and in group therapy for six months. She arrived at the group session very angry at the other group members, because they had agreed to call each other up and go out together, but no one called her. She told the group the following:

'You really can't trust anybody! You guys only talk, but deep down you are just as irresponsible and bad as everybody else! I don't know if it is worth having therapy if people are so comfortable in their ways that they don't care about other people's feelings. I won't make any more plans with you again!'

Various group members tried to justify why nobody called her, but to all of them R replied with a growing fury, without accepting any excuses or conciliatory attempts. At this point the therapist made a double from the group telling R how powerless they felt because of her refusal to accept anything that they were offering her.

R became even angrier, saying that now the group was the one to feel sorry about and she became the bad one, when in reality the situation was exactly the other way around. Then the therapist stood next to her and, taking on her bodily position, said the following in a low voice:

'I would like so much to be understood, and not to be accused…I feel so sad…I wanted so much to be with you guys during the past week…everything has gone wrong! And now…everything is getting even worse…I don't know how to fix it…I am feeling more and more alone!'

As a result of the double, the client started to cry and became able to change her attitude towards the group; at the same time, the group also managed to get closer and talk to her.

The mirror technique can be very useful in allowing one to see from a distance the power struggles involved in the interactions, as well as the resulting psychodynamics. The therapist can formulate a synthesis of what was shown in the scene, accentuating aspects that the client may still not be able to realize. It can be seen as an *in loco* reinterpretation of the facts that were interpreted differently by the client.

Case example: L

L, a 20-year-old client, is becoming an alcoholic and she is getting more and more involved with hard drugs. According to her, she is not able to resist drugs when she knows that there is the possibility of getting them. However, after using them, she feels very bad and regrets allowing herself to take them.

Starting off with a scene in which she gives in to drugs, L recalls another scene where she was four years old, and being alone in the house, felt sad and abandoned. While playing with a ball all alone, she thought that if she hurt herself, her parents would have to come home and take care of her. Following this thought, she threw herself against the wall with all her might, injuring her head and starting to bleed.

Her parents were notified and they returned immediately to help her. Even though she was in pain, L felt happy: her parents were worried about her and stayed with her. It wasn't such a big price to pay after all!

After marking all the characters with cushions, the therapist asks her to step out of the scene and observe it from the outside. The therapist encourages L to observe from her adult role what is happening to the little girl.

'Look what is happening to that little girl. She is learning that by hurting herself she can get attention, and she is going to carry on doing this in her adult life. Her ability for self-destruction will continue growing: she will get involved in car accidents, she will consume great amounts of alcohol, she will start to take harder and harder drugs...Do you think this is what she really wants? What do you think she needed before she started to hurt herself?'

L is sadly watching the little girl, saying that she needed love and affection, but her parents were unable to give it to her spontaneously. The therapist asks her (as the adult) to hold this deprived little girl and see if they still want to carry on with her self-aggression and self-destruction; see if they still think that this is a reasonable price to pay for love and attention.

Holding in her arms the cushion representing the little girl, L speaks to her affectionately, and tells her that this is not what she wanted and that they should find another way to get love and affection; this would take time however, because she didn't know how to do it differently.

Mirroring is therefore a privileged place for insights, both for the client and the therapist. It is important that the therapist follows accurately the material brought by the client and that he doesn't distort it with his own personal material or his theories.

The technique of surplus reality can also be very valuable when working with borderline clients, because it may allow them to catch a glimpse (even if only in fantasy) of the necessary solutions of the various dead-end situations in which they often find themselves.

Case example: B

B, a 27-year-old client, has been in individual and group therapy for four years. He complains of professional dissatisfaction, because he always ends up having to take on more responsibility than his work partner. He feels unable to discuss this matter with his partner without internally becoming resentful and aggressive, while outwardly presenting a submissive and powerless attitude.

He enacts a scene presenting this reaction in front of his partner. The therapist asks him if there was any other situation in his life where he felt that same way. Promptly, B recalls an old scene (already known by the therapist): following the suicide of his mother, he is desperately trying to please his father, even though he feels the unjustness of his situation. In the absence of anyone who would care for him or he could trust, the weak and helpless six-year-old child does not have an alternative.

The therapist suggests that B invents the parents that he would like to have. Visibly delighted, the client chooses two group members, whom he likes a lot, to play the role of his ideal – caring, affectionate and encouraging – parents. He spends a good deal of time 'enjoying' his parents, coaching them until he feels fully satisfied.

Then the therapist suggests returning to the scene with his work partner, but this time with the support of these 'ideal parents', who will stand behind the client cheering for him. B looks at his partner and looks at his 'parents', who look back at him tenderly; his body posture becomes more erect and he talks calmly with his partner:

'I have been very unhappy for some time with how things go in the company. I think we need to talk things through properly, because I am thinking of breaking up the partnership.'

In the following session B tells the group that his 'artificial parents' seem to have injected him with a strength that is helping him not only in solving his issues with his partner, but also some other problematic life situations.

A very useful technique when working with the client's aggression is the concretization of anger, combined with the interpolation of a metaphor that symbolizes the concretized product. Cukier (1995) has described in detail this work of character interpolation, demonstrating that through the relaxation of the client's intra-psychic area, reactive and defensive roles can be more easily experienced by the client, and these can be highlighted from the rest of the personality.

Case example: A

A, a 43-year-old woman, has been in individual therapy for two years. She complains of a debilitating jealousy towards her husband and frequent aggressive outbursts triggered by situations in which she feels insecure as a woman. In one of the sessions, she sets up a scene of her husband coming home late in the night. The therapist suggests the following to her:

'Show me without words, only with your body, how you are feeling.'

The client lifts her arms and curls her fingers as if they were claws, and flashes her teeth as if they were fangs, giving the impression of a beast. The therapist asks her to exaggerate her tension. The client tenses up completely, looking like a monster contorted by rage. The therapist allows her to experience this bodily tension for a while, and then assertively suggests:

'Now I want you to find a character, a character from a story or a film, any character who may feel like this.'

'Anything?' asks the client.

'Yes, the first thing that comes to your mind, anything.'

'A tellurian woman' she answers firmly.

'What are you like, tellurian woman?' asks the therapist curiously.

'I am half woman, a sensual woman, and half beast; like a jaguar with its fangs ready to rip its prey apart.'

The therapist carries on interviewing this tellurian woman, trying to find out her story, when she first appeared, what kind of power she has, etc.

Following this role play, the therapist invites the client to return to her own role, and tell when and why she needed to create this tellurian woman inside herself.

The client promptly recalls a scene when she was five years old, and was taken to a psychologist against her will. As soon as she got there, she began to kick, scream and, on one occasion, she even broke a window. The tellurian woman was her childhood defence that she had created against the disempowerment she felt for being treated as crazy. She became 'crazy' in revenge for being considered 'crazy'.

The metaphor of the 'Tellurian Woman' was used for many sessions and a collage was made to concretize it. It became a jargon between the client and therapist that was used every time they wanted to refer to A's aggressive defence reactions, which deep inside caused her more damage than defence.

We believe that when a borderline client begins to understand the defensive nature of his aggressive parts, these can acquire dignity. The client will stop identifying with them, and will start to search actively for more appropriate ways of defending himself. Concretization and the interpolation of metaphors can be extremely useful for this purpose.

Finally, we would like to make some brief comments regarding the technique of role reversal. Experiencing the role of the other allows the client to absorb aspects of the relationship that he had not known, and it also enables the therapist to gain a more integral view of the psychodynamic process.

When investigating childhood scenes with borderline clients, we often come across an 'other', an abusive adult. It is important for the client to receive support in connection with the experience of abuse; however, it is also equally important for him to rescue some positive aspect from these primary relationships, without denying the abuse and its emotional consequences.

Case example: S

S, a 28-year-old client, was systematically beaten with a wooden rod during his childhood. In the role of his mother, he tells the therapist that she was also beaten during her childhood with a copper wire. When beating her son with the wooden rod, her intention was she to give him the same education but to hurt him less.

By discovering the real intention of the abusive parent, this client managed to rescue a small but kind aspect of his mother, which was in some way comforting for him.

Conclusions

Working with borderline clients represents a constant challenge for the therapist. The pain resulting from a childhood that was lacking basic care and validation will strongly mark the relationships of these clients, making them suspicious, demanding, scheming, and continuously dissatisfied. Finding the balance between attitudes of acceptance, support and validation on the one hand, and the structuring boundaries of reality on the other, is a difficult task for the therapist.

The seductive role of the 'saviour' (trying to fulfil the client's enormous needs), or 'blaming the victim' (making the client responsible for the failure of therapy), are traps that are constantly present during the therapeutic work. The 'emotional skin' that can help the client to contain and organize his feelings, is built up through a creative therapeutic relationship by implanting small 'skin grafts' bit by bit, giving these clients a protective shell and covering, so they can grow and develop with dignity.

Notes

1   Originally published under the title: 'Eu te odeio...por favor não me abandones! – O paciente borderline e o psicodrama'. In R. Cukier (1998) *Sobrevivência Emocional – As Dores da Infância Revividas no Drama Adulto [Emotional Survival – Re-living Childhood Pain in the Drama of the Adult]*. São Paulo: Ágora, p.73–98.

2   Millon (1987) suggested the term cycloid personality to emphasize the instability of behaviour and mood that he considered to be central in these conditions. According to him, the borderline pattern results from a deterioration of other, less severe personality patterns. He believes that the borderline personality can develop in various ways, since the clients' clinical histories are different.

3   The term 'para-suicidal behaviour' was introduced by Kreisman in 1977 to describe intentional, but non-fatal, self-destructive behaviour (self-mutilation, drug abuse, self-inflicted burns, suicidal thoughts). It also includes suicidal gestures and manipulations. Para-suicidal, however, is a more appropriate and less pejorative term than manipulator. The difficulty in treating these individuals makes one frequently blame the clients, which obviously does not help them.

4   Falivene Alves (1995) pointed out that in every group (for example the family) there are sociometric factors that represent 'external authorization' for an individual's behaviour. Exposed to this power, each person will develop a corresponding

'internal authorization'. In extremely damaged clients this internal authorization may be so fragile that they will be extremely dependent on external permissions. The equilibrium between the external and the internal authority represents the basis of a true authority. When being permissive and validating the client's emotions and behaviours, the therapist functions as a new external authority aiming to reinforce the client's internal authority.

5   Miller (1979) has shown that a large number of therapists come from families where they were asked to be the 'good children' who help their parents.

14

Sociometry
A new way to calculate the indices of the perceptive test[1]

Antonio Ferrara

Objective

Over the years, the sociometric test created by Moreno has gone through many modifications. When used for therapeutic purposes – in its actual form – it is very valuable; this value consists in the indices obtained through the evaluation of the *perceptive test* (these indices are: the perception index, emission index, tele index, and the index of group tele). Bustos (1979) proposed the use of graphic representations in order to calculate these indices; a method that is useful for those people who have a better understanding of these graphical representations. This chapter aims to present an alternative way of representing these indices, by grouping the data in a table that can be read more easily.

The importance of perception

In order to understand the importance of the perceptive test and its indices, we will need to review the concept of tele from the perspective of the communication theory and the information based on which the sociometric test is evaluated.

The concept of tele from the perspective of the communication theory

> To understand communication, we need to look at tele as a relational concept, indicating the flow of messages that shapes the dynamics of the encounter. When defining tele, Moreno talks about the perception of distance; however, distance is just one characteristic of the dynamics

of a relationship. Another characteristic would be emission, these two characteristics representing two directions of the relationship. (Bustos 1979, p.48)

Communication theory describes three different components in any communication process: the emitter, the message and the receiver:

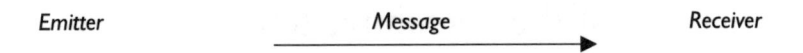

Emitter — Message → Receiver

This theory also postulates that without an emitter and a receiver communication cannot exist, and if these two elements exist it is impossible not to have communication, because a message will also always exist between them (the absence of a message is also a message in itself). In this sense Watzlawick stated that 'we can postulate a meta-communicational axiom regarding communication: it is not possible not to communicate' (Watzlawick, Beavin and Jackson 1981, p.47).

We can say then, that in the communication process the messages emitted by the emitter are received by the receiver and that for this to happen they (emitter and receiver) need to be in relation. As Watzlawick said: 'any communication implies an engagement and therefore it defines the concept of the emitter in relation to the receiver' (Watzlawick *et al.* 1981, p.47).

Let's examine the following two communications:

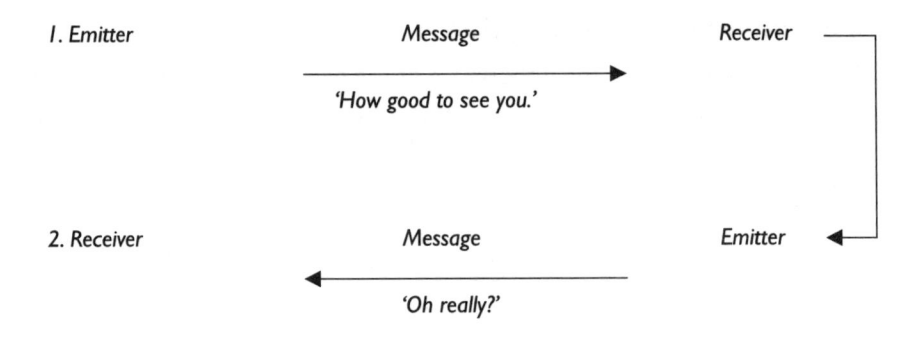

1. Emitter — Message → Receiver
'How good to see you.'

2. Receiver ← Message — Emitter
'Oh really?'

Even in a simple example like this we can find different possibilities for the 'failure' of the communication:

- The first possibility would be that the emitter has no real desire to encounter the other person, but for some reason he wants to seem nice and says: 'How good to see you.' In this case the emitter doesn't emit a correct message, or in other words, what he says is not congruent with what he feels; in the terminology used by Bustos (1979), he would be a *faulty emitter*.

- The other possibility is that the emitter has a genuine desire to encounter the other person and is really expressing what he feels when saying 'How good to see you.' On the other hand, though, it is the receiver who finds it difficult to perceive that another person may be interested in him: he receives the emitter's message with suspicion and is reluctant to accept that the other person is really pleased to meet (encounter) him. He responds sceptically: 'Oh really?' In this case, we talk about a *faulty receiver*.

We could bring many other examples of faulty emitters and faulty receivers, or correct emitters and correct receivers, these latter being the other two 'sociometric character types', defined by Bustos (1979, p.49). What is important at this point is that the messages emitted in a communication process can be wrongly emitted and/or wrongly received. Certainly neither of these should happen in a *tele relationship*. In order to verify the existence of a tele relationship, we need to examine the following four aspects in the communication of two people:

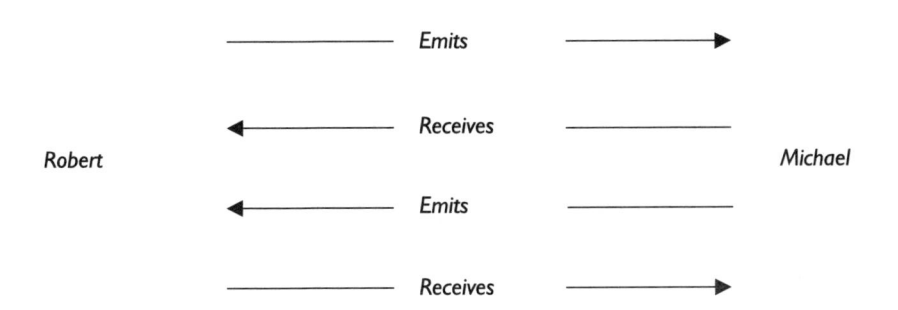

```
                ——————— Emits    ——————▶
                ◀——————— Receives   ———————
Robert                                              Michael
                ◀——————— Emits    ———————
                ——————— Receives  ——————▶
```

In other words, we will need to verify whether the message emitted by Robert is emitted correctly and is also received that way (correctly) by Michael; and, at the same time, whether the message emitted by Michael is emitted correctly and it is also received correctly by Robert.

When applying the sociometric test, we will need to evaluate the answers (responses) written down by each group member, regarding his/her communications with the others. Having the responses of each of the group member, we can compare these. This is our next topic.

The information based on which the sociometric test is evaluated

According to my definition of sociometry, social systems consist of preferences or in other words, attraction–rejection–neutrality' (Moreno 1934, p.xlii).

> It is difficult for us to stay emotionally neutral in relation to the people with whom we constantly come into contact.... In the same way it rarely happens that the others will express feelings of emotional neutrality toward us.... Affective attraction and repulsion between two people will influence a whole series of social behaviours such as susceptibility to influence and identification, imitation and aggression, the use of power, the formation of groups, social perception, etc. (Rodrigues 1977, p.319)

When applying a sociometric test, we basically propose to analyse the group by asking each group member to answer the following two questions:

- 'Whom would you choose to…(criterion)?'
- 'Who do you think would choose you to…(criterion)?'

In order to answer these questions group members also need to have a *sociometric criterion* based on which they can make their choices within the group. In order to assure that these choices are made in an adequate and possibly free manner, the criterion for these choices needs to be discussed by the group, it needs to emerge from the group. It is 'the responsibility of the director to apply the test only after the group has chosen a sound criterion and discussed all its specifications' (Bustos 1979, p. 5) Actually, this group discussion around the sociometric criteria also serves as a warm-up for the application of the sociometric test.

As an example, Bustos (1979, p.76) presents the following sociometric criterion:

- With whom would you choose to *do a dramatic exercise?*
- Who do you think would choose to *do a dramatic exercise with* you?

According to Bustos, 'a human being has many criteria as well as many actions' (1979, p.34). When applying the sociometric test, each group member will need to make his/her own choices and formulate his/her answers, according to the following three categories:

- People whom I would choose (and I think that would choose me) *positively.*
- People towards whom I would choose to be *indifferent* (and I think they would choose to be *indifferent* towards me).
- People whom I would choose (and I think they would choose me) *negatively.*

We ask each group member to make their choices in a *hierarchical* way within these three categories, that is, to choose a *most positive* person, a *second most positive* person and so on, applying this hierarchical structure also to the *negative* and *indifferent* choices.

The two questions mentioned above are aimed at investigating different aspects of a relationship:

- 'Whom would you choose to...?' This is an *objective test* that allows the investigation of the external group ('the group that can be viewed by an observer' [Bustos 1979, p.46]); the response to this question is a clear indication of the choices made by a group member in relation to the others; it is 'the real image of the group'; it is an objective test based on the 'dynamics of choosing' and is called 'extrovert'.
- 'Who do you think would choose you to...?' This is a *perceptive test*, which allows the investigation 'of the internal representation of the group within each one of its members', or the 'internal group'; it is a perceptive test based on the 'dynamics of social perception' and is called 'introvert'.

So, after applying the test, the sociometrist has in his hands a certain amount of answers given to these two questions. These responses will constitute the base for the evaluation of the sociometric test. Now he can start making some comparisons, such as:

- If A has chosen B as second in his positive choices, how will B choose A? Will he have the same preference or choice (that is, will A also be in second place among B's positive choices)? In the case of the choices of A and B matching, we talk about an equal choice or *mutuality*; in the case of the two choices not matching, we talk about *incongruence*.

- If X thinks that he is the most positively chosen group member by Y, the sociometrist can check if this really matches with the actual choices made by Y (of course, only if he has the relevant answer from Y).

We can make a whole series of comparisons between the responses which we obtained, resulting in information regarding the mutuality, incongruence, etc. of the choices. The different possible comparisons are described in detail by Bustos (1979); within this chapter I would like to focus mainly on what he said regarding the perceptive test.

When comparing the answers we can observe *distortions* or differences between 'the group as it really exists' and 'the group as each member thinks (perceives) it exists':

1. *The group as it really exists*: this information is obtained based on the answers that each member gave to the question, 'Whom would you choose?' It reflects the real feelings of each group member, expressed in their choices related to the others.

2. *The group as each group member thinks (perceives) it exists*: this information is obtained based on the answers the group members gave to the question, 'Who do you think would choose you?' In order to respond to this question, the group member needs to role reverse with all the other group members and try to discover their feelings in relation to him. This question no longer deals with the group as it really exists (and could be seen by an observer), but with the 'internal representation of the group within each one of its members' (Bustos 1979, p.46).

Distortions and differences which appear when comparing the group as it exists and the group as each member thinks (perceives) that it exists occur as a result of the fact that 'nobody sees the group as it really is; the emotions of the individual will always alter the perception of the group from how it really is' (Bustos 1979, p.46).

Bustos has pointed out the risk that some group members will not emit correctly, but in order to make the evaluation they will be considered as correct-emitters. This, however, will be diluted if we consider that each member when analysed will be compared with all the others in the group; among these group members there will be good and bad (faulty) emitters, and this is why we refer to the group as 'average'.

After he has applied the sociometric test, the sociometrist will have a series of answers to the questions: 'Whom would you choose to…(criterion)?' and 'Who do you think would choose you to…(criterion)?'

Having this information will allow the comparison of the *image of the group* existing in a certain group member with the *actually existing group*, quantifying the existing distortion between this image and the actual (real) group. Through the evaluation of the perceptive test we can also verify how each group member is situated in his relationship with every other group member, identifying his 'communicational responsibility' in the establishment of tele relations.

How can we calculate the indices of the perceptive test?

The graphic representation developed by Bustos

> In order to evaluate the perceptive aspect of the test, we draw a circle for each group member and divide it into two halves. In the upper semi-circle we will note the perception of each person; while in the lower semi-circle we'll note how the person was really chosen, or in other words the objective observations of the others. (Bustos 1979, p.47)

In order to exemplify this method, I will present a protocol of a sociometric test carried out by Bustos. The protocol itself (the questions given to the group members and their responses) and the corresponding graphic representations can be found in Bustos's book (1979, pp.86–99). Figure 14.1 (p.236) presents the diagram of a group member whom he calls C.

234   SAMBADRAMA

```
PERCEPTIVE TEST*
(of the group member who is being
evaluated)

OBJECTIVE TEST**
(of the other group members, in their
relation to the evaluated
group member)
```

Perceptive test: information obtained from C in response to the question 'Who do you think would choose you...?'

Objective test: information obtained from the other group members in response to the question 'Whom would you choose to...?' in relation to C

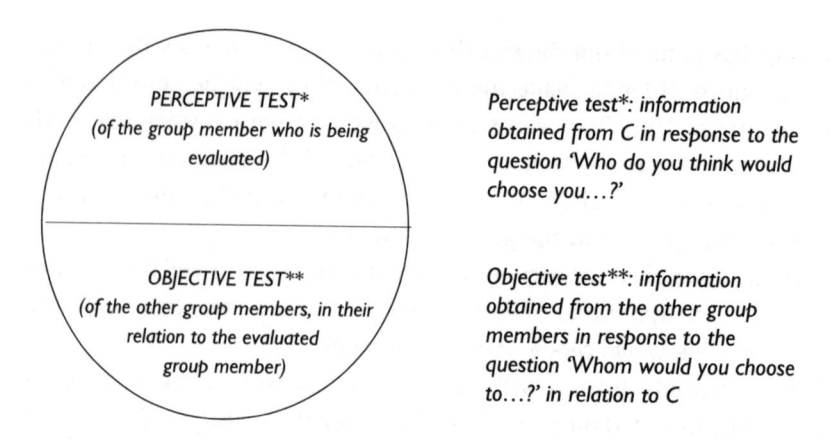

Figure 14.1 The graphic representation of C. (Source: Bustos 1979, p.86, reproduced with permission)

In the next step Bustos divides the upper semi-circle into as many segments as there are members of the group minus one (corresponding to C who is being evaluated). Every choice is tinted, separate tints representing the positive, negative and neutral choices. Figure 14.2 is the graphic representation for the perceptive test of group member C.

Key

■ (+) Positive choices

▨ (±) Neutral choices

▧ (–) Negative choices

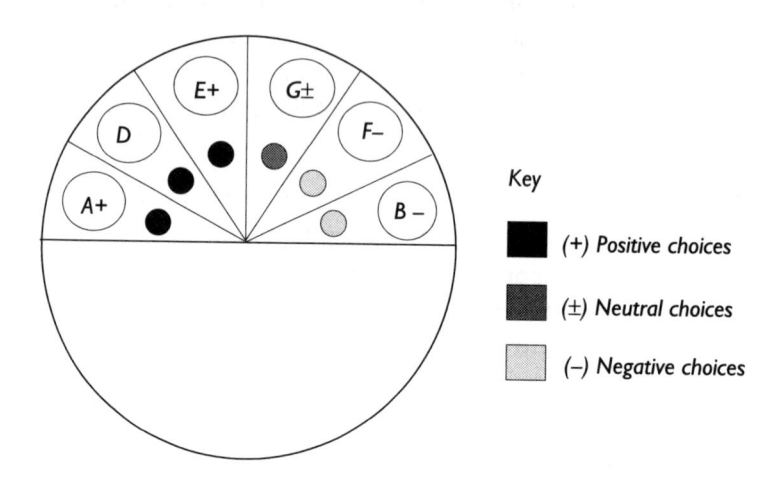

Figure 14.2 The perceptive test of group member C (Source: Bustos 1979, p.86, reproduced with permission)

It is important to observe the following:

1. The group has seven members; C does not figure in this graphic representation (Figure 14.2), because it represents his own choices.

2. The group members are placed in the diagram from left to right in function of the choices made by C (in accordance with his perception of the other group members).

Positive   Neutral   Negative

On the left (originally marked with blue, generally used for positive choices) are those group members whom C thinks would choose him positively (A, D and E); to their right is G (originally marked with green) whom C considers to be indifferent towards him; and finally on the right hand side of the diagram are F and B (originally marked with red – a colour used for negative choices) whom are perceived by C as choosing him negatively.

All the information presented so far refers to how C perceives the choices of the other group members in relation to him. It is a hypothesis made by C, an internal representation of the group from C's perspective, in relation to himself.

In the lower semi-circle, using the same tint-coding, we will represent how the person (C) was really perceived (chosen) by the other group members, or in other words the perspective of the other group members (see Figure 14.3, p.236). In both the segments of the upper and lower semi-circle we will include the initials used for the group members, marking with an asterisk those where the perception of the analysed person corresponds to the objective perception of the other.

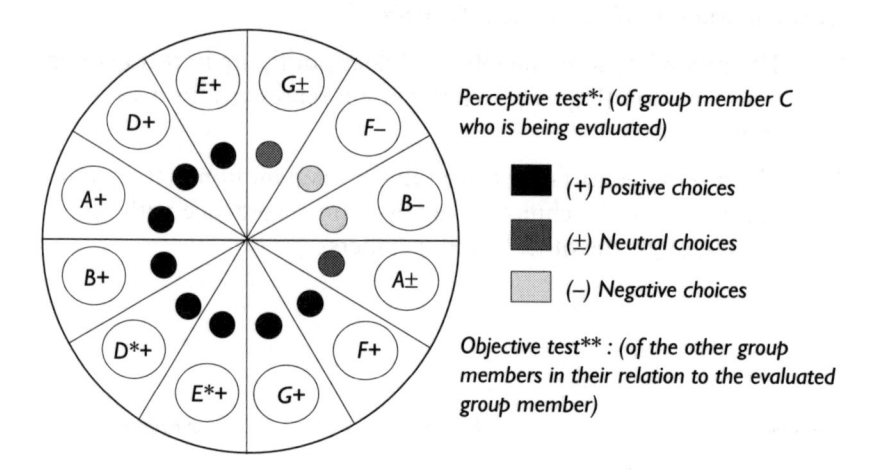

Figure 14.3 The graphic representation of both the perceptive and the objective test for group member C (Source: Bustos 1979, p.86, reproduced with permission)

The lower semi-circle contains the answers of the other group members for the question 'Whom would you choose?' Based on this graphic representation, Bustos describes the following comparisons.

The upper semi-circle shows that C thinks that A would choose him positively; but is his hypothesis correct? Looking at the lower semi-circle we can see that this hypothesis is not correct: in reality A is neutral (indifferent) towards C. This means that C's internal representation of A does not correspond to the reality: he wasn't chosen by A as he imagined. We can assume two explanations for this discrepancy:

- C does not perceive the messages emitted by A correctly (C is a faulty-receiver)
- A does not emit his indifference correctly (A is a faulty-emitter).

But which one of these two assumptions is right? At this moment we cannot know, but if we carry on with the analysis we will, we hope, find the answer.

Bustos continues to compare the other hypotheses of C (the perception of C) with the answers given by the other group members in relation to him. He finds out that C has made correct assumptions only in relation to D and E (he assumed that they would choose him positively, which corresponds to the reality). These responses are marked with an asterisk. 'Based on the perceptive test we can calculate a perception index that measures the perceptive ability of a person. This index can be calculated by relating the number of concurrencies to the number of the possibilities (the number of group members minus one)' (Bustos 1979, p.48).

In the above graphic representation (Figure 14.3) we can see that C has six possibilities (there are six other group members). Out of these six he only got two of his assumptions right. This means that C's *perception index* is 2/6. (It is important to note that this index is not simply calculated based on the number of corresponding colour segments; in the upper semi-circle there are three positive segments while in the lower semi-circle there are five – this however does not mean that there are three concurrencies.)

This already gives us some indication in response to the above question, whether C is a faulty-receiver or A is a faulty-emitter. It seems that C is the one who has some sort of problem with his perception. A more concrete indication would be if we could also verify the *emission index* of A.

Bustos carries on with further comparisons for all the other group members. He prepares the same graphic representation for the other six group members as well, in the upper semi-circle marking the responses of the perceptive test given by the analysed person, while in the lower semi-circle the objective responses of the other group members in relation to the one being analysed.

Thus he obtains seven circular diagrams, one for each of the group members (Figure 14.4, p.238). Having all seven diagrams available, we now have the conditions to calculate the emission indices for all seven group members.

> The ability to emit messages is evaluated by counting how many times the person in question had been marked with an asterisk in the lower semi-circle of the diagrams belonging to the other group members. (Bustos 1979, p.49)

In case of C we can observe that there are five diagrams where there is an asterisk next to his name in the lower semi-circle: B, D, E, F and G. This means that his positive messages are concurrent with the internal representations made by B, D, E, F and G. These five group members perceive exactly what C emits (a positive choice), because they assumed (perceived) that C would choose them positively.

Given that besides C there are six other group members, the *emission index* of C will be 5/6; a good index.

238   SAMBADRAMA

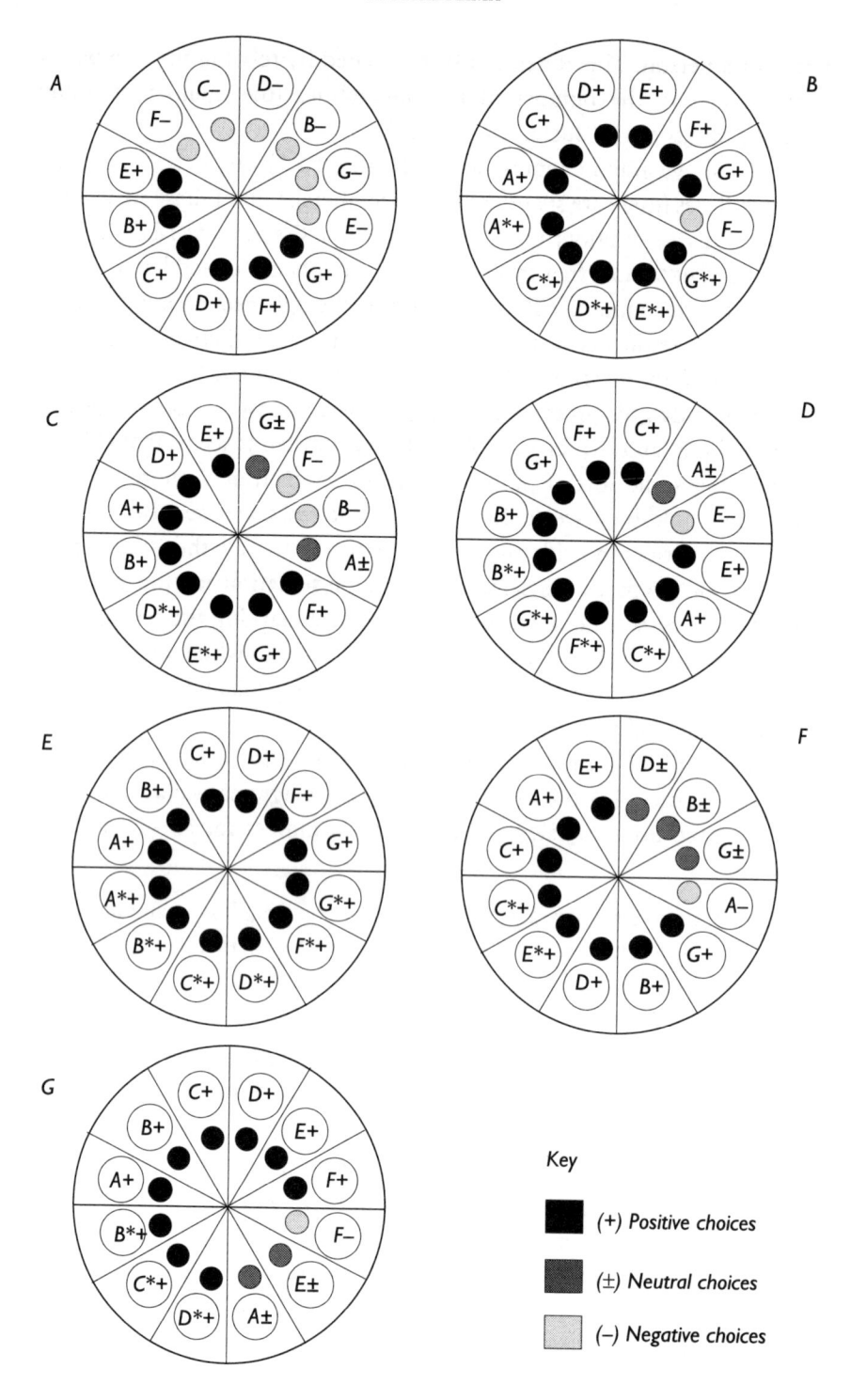

Figure 14.4 The graphic representations for all seven group members (Source: Bustos 1979, p.86, reproduced with permission)

Having had calculated both the *perception index* (2/6) and the *emission index* (5/6) for C, now we are able to calculate his *tele index*:

> tele – in its dynamicity – implies both emission and perception. The *tele index* evaluates communication globally and tells us the degree of adaptation of the individual in relation to himself and the group of which he is a part (Bustos 1979, p.51).

The *tele index* is calculated as the simple arithmetic average of the other two indices (perception and emission index), keeping the common denominator, which is the same for both indices. In case of C the tele index will be calculated in the following way:

Perception index	Emission index	Calculation	Tele index
2/6	5/6	(2+5):2/6	3.5/6

Even though C has a 'low' perception index, his emission index is high and this fact elevates his tele index.

This will take us back to the question asked before: in relation to A, is C a faulty-receptor or a faulty-emitter? Our last assumption was that C has some sort of perception problem. This is partially confirmed if we take into consideration that C has a low (2/6) perception index, but for a more conclusive answer regarding the relationship of A and C we will also need to analyse the perception and emission indices of A.

Based on the above presented diagrams and following the same rationale, A would have the following indices:

Perception index	Emission index	Calculation	Tele index
0/6	2/6	(0+2):2/6	1/6

We can see that A has an emission index of 2/6 which is considered low; so in the relation of A and C besides the 'faulty' perception of C, the 'faulty' emission of A also has an important role.

Now let us take a look at their tele indices: C=3.5/6; A=1/6. Based on these figures we can assume that C has a better ability (capacity) to establish tele relationships than A. It is the tele index that will help us understand their relationship. In his book, Bustos makes a detailed analysis of these two group members, evaluating also the mutuality and incongruence of their choices. He also compares the tele indices of these two group members with the *index of group tele,* which is 3.1.

The index of group tele represents 'the quantity of tele that the group contains' (Bustos 1979, p.52), and it is the arithmetical average of all the tele indices within the group. In the group used as an example:

Tele index	Index of group tele
A 1/6	
B 4/6	
C 3.5/6	
D 4/6	(1+4+3.5+4+4.5+2+3):7/6 = 3.1/6
E 4.5/6	
F 2/6	
G 3/6	

This is the graphic representation proposed by Bustos for the evaluation of perception (perception index, emission index, tele index and the index of group tele). It is called 'graphic', because it uses circular graphs (charts) to represent the information regarding each group member.

The tabular form of calculation: a new way of representation

In order to simplify matters for people who find it easier to read data out of tables, in the following I will present a tabular way of calculating the indices of the perceptive test.

Based on the answers given by the group members to the perceptive test (internal group) and objective test (external group), this new way of representation consists in the elaboration of a table. Within this table, information (data) is arranged as presented in Figure 14.5.

This table will have as many rows and columns as the number of group members and we add to it:

- three more columns (one for the heading, one for the perception index and one for the tele index)
- two more rows (one for the headings and one for the emission index).

SOCIOMETRY

OBJECTIVE TEST (Whom would you choose?)

PERCEPTIVE TEST

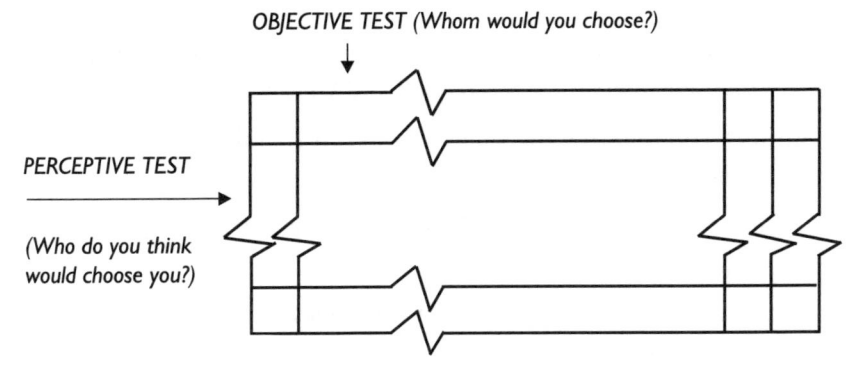

(Who do you think would choose you?)

Figure 14.5 Setting out the table for the tabular calculation of indices

So, in case of a group consisting of seven members (as in our example), the table will have:

- 7+3=10 columns, and
- 7+2=9 rows (Table 14.1).

Table 14.1 Drawing up the table for the tabular way of calculation									
Perceptive evaluation	*A*	*B*	*C*	*D*	*E*	*F*	*G*	*Perception index*	*Tele index*
A	X								
B		X							
C			X						
D				X					
E					X				
F						X			
G							X		
Emission index							X	(*)

We can observe that:

- the first row and the first column are used for including the group members (A, B, C, D, E, F and G) as well as the headings
- in the bottom row the values of the emission index will be included
- in the second column from the right the values of the perception index will be included
- in the first column on the right the values of the tele index will be included
- while in the right bottom, marked with (*) we will include the index of group tele
- since group members do not make choices about themselves, crosses are placed diagonally in the table.

Table 14.2 Dividing the rows for the inclusion of the results of the perceptive (1) and the objective (2) test

Perceptive evaluation	A	B	C	D	E	F	G	Perception index	Tele index
A1	X								
2									
B1		X							
2									
C1			X						
2									
D1				X					
2									
E1					X				
2									
F1						X			
2									
G1							X		
2									

In the next step, each row corresponding for the group members will be divided in two lines - one for the results of the perceptive test, and one for the result of the objective test (Table 14.2). Now the table is ready for the inclusion of the data.

Filling in the table

In the first line of each horizontal row we will include the results of the *perceptive test* for each group member (corresponding to the internal group as seen by each group member). In other words, these are the responses to the question 'Who do you think would choose you?' (placed in the upper semi-circle in Bustos's representation). Table 14.3 is a representation of the group in Bustos's example. Based on the great number of positive signs, we can already notice that the group has a great expectation to be chosen positively (the question was: 'Who do you think would choose you?').

Table 14.3 Including the results of the perceptive test										
Perceptive evaluation	A	B	C	D	E	F	G	Perception index	Tele index
A 1 2	X	−	−	−	+	−	−		
B 1 2	+	X	+	+	+	+	+		
C 1 2	+	−	X	+	+	−	±		
D 1 2	±	+	+	X	−	+	+		
E 1 2	+	+	+	+	X	+	+		
F 1 2	+	±	+	±	+	X	±		
G 1 2	+	+	+	+	+	+	X		
Emission index								X	(*)

In the second line of each horizontal row now we will include the results of the *objective test* (these correspond to the external group) – see Table 14.4. In other words, these are the responses given to the question 'Whom would you choose?' (placed in the lower semi-circle in Bustos's representation). Keeping in mind that in this second line we include responses to the question 'Whom would you choose?' we can observe that the group has made numerous positive choices. Having been filled in with the necessary information, the table now is ready for the calculation of the indices.

Table 14.4 Including the results of the objective test										
Perceptive evaluation	A	B	C	D	E	F	G	Perception index	Tele index
A1	X	–	–	–	+	–	–		
2		+	+	+	–	+	+		
B1	+	X	+	+	+	+	+		
2	+		+	+	+	–	+		
C1	+	–	X	+	+	–	±		
2	±	+		+	+	+	+		
D1	±	+	+	X	–	+	+		
2	+	+	+		+	+	+		
E1	+	+	+	+	X	+	+		
2	+	+	+	+		+	+		
F1	+	±	+	±	+	X	±		
2	–	+	+	+	+		+		
G1	+	+	+	+	+	+	X		
2	±	+	+	+	±	–			
Emission index								X	(*)

How to calculate the perception index?

In order to calculate the perception index for a certain group member, we will need to check that in the row corresponding to this member, how many signs correspond (concur) between the first and the second line of the row. The number of concurrences will be the numerator of the perception index, while the denominator will be the number of group members minus one. Table 14.5 shows how to calculate the perception index for group member C. We use the same rationale to calculate the perception index for the rest of the group members.

Table 14.5 Calculating the perception index for group member C									
Perceptive evaluation	A	B	C	D	E	F	G	Perception index
C1	+	–	X	+	+	–	±	2/6
2	±	+		+	+	+	+	
Concurrence:	no	no	X	yes	yes	no	no	

How many concurrences?   2
Number of group members minus one: 6
Perception index for C: 2/6

How to calculate the emission index?

In order to calculate the emission index, we will need to count the concurrences in the vertical column corresponding to a certain group member. In the case of group member C, we will proceed according to Table 14.6. We use the same rationale in order to calculate the emission index for the other group members.

Table 14.6 Calculating the emission index for group member C

Perceptive evaluation	C	Perception index	Tele index	Concurrence
A1	−			No
2	+			
B1	+			Yes
2	+			
C1	X			X
2				
D1	+			Yes
2	+			
E1	+			Yes
2	+			
F1	+			Yes
2	+			
G1	+			Yes
2	+			
Emission index	5/6			

How many concurrences? 5
Number of group members minus one: 6
Emission index for C: 5/6

How to calculate the tele index and the index of group tele?

After having calculated the perception and emission indexes for all group members, our table will look as shown in Table 14.7.

Table 14.7 Emission and perception indices for all group members

Perception evaluation	A	B	C	D	E	F	G	Perception index	Tele index
A1	X	−	−	−	+	−	−	0/6	
2		+	+	+	−	+	+		
B1	+	X	+	+	+	+	+	5/6	
2	+		+	+	+	−	+		
C1	+	−	X	+	+	−	±	2/6	
2	±	+		+	+	+	+		
D1	±	+	+	X	−	+	+	4/6	
2	+	+	+		+	+	+		
E1	+	+	+	+	X	+	+	6/6	
2	+	+	+	+		+	+		
F1	+	±	+	±	+	X	±	2/6	
2	−	+	+	+	+		+		
G1	+	+	+	+	+	+	X	3/6	
2	±	+	+	+	±	−			
Emission index	2/6	3/6	5/6	4/6	3/6	2/6	3/6	X	(*)

To calculate the tele index for each group member we will use the same formula as Bustos: we'll calculate the arithmetic average of the perception and emission index, including the result into the right hand side column of the table. For the calculation of the index of group tele we will also use the same formula as Bustos, the result being marked in the bottom row of the far right-hand column, marked with (*). Let us now calculate the tele index for each group calculating the tele index for each group member, based on the following table:

Table 14.8 Calculating the tele index for each group member				
Group member	Perception index	Emitter index	Calculation	Tele index
A	0/6	2/6	(0+2):2/6	1/6
B	5/6	3/6	(5+3):2/6	4/6
C	2/6	5/6	(2+5):2/6	3.5/6
D	4/6	4/6	(4+4):2/6	4/6
E	6/6	3/6	(6+3):2/6	4.5/6
F	2/6	2/6	(2+2):2/6	2/6

After including these indices in our table, the index of group tele is calculated in the following way: (1+4+3.5+4+4.5+2+3):7/6=3.1/6. This result is also included in the table. Now the table contains all results and indices (Table 14.9). For better visualization the table can also be colour-coded.

Conclusions

We can observe that in the tabular form of representation the reading and comparison of the information is straightforward, simply by comparing line 1 and 2 in each row, and in order to do this it is not necessary to consult all the separate graphic representations. Furthermore, in this tabular representation there is also a separate box for all the indices (perception index, emission index, tele index and index of group tele).

The tabular representation also allows a better overview of all the information at the same time, without needing to consult separately all the different charts for each individual (group member).

Note

1 Originally published under the title: 'Sociometria: uma nova forma para calcular indices do teste perceptual.' *Revista Brasileira de Psicodrama I*, 2, 1990, pp.29–56.

Table 14.9 Calculating the tele index for each group member and the index of group tele

Perception evaluation	A	B	C	D	E	F	G	Perception index	Tele index
A1	X	−	−	−	+	−	−	0/6	1/6
2		+	+	+	−	+	+		
B1	+	X	+	+	+	+	+	5/6	4/6
2	+		+	+	+	−	+		
C1	+	−	X	+	+	−	±	2/6	3.5/6
2	±	+		+	+	+	+		
D1	±	+	+	X	−	+	+	4/6	4/6
2	+	+	+		+	+	+		
E1	+	+	+	+	X	+	+	6/6	4.5/6
2	+	+	+	+		+	+		
F1	+	±	+	±	+	X	±	2/6	2/6
2	−	+	+	+	+		+		
G1	+	+	+	+	+	+	X	3/6	3/6
2	±	+	+	+	±	−			
Emission index	2/6	3/6	5/6	4/6	3/6	2/6	3/6	X	3.1/6

15

Video-psychodrama and tele-psychodrama
The research of a Morenian dream[1]

Ronaldo Pamplona da Costa

Historical background

From very early on in his professional career, Moreno showed an interest in the media and means of communication, such as radio, cinema and television. As early as the 1920s, while studying medicine in Vienna, Moreno (together with his brother-in-law) had developed a sound recording device to reproduce music and voice. After he emmigrated to the US, Moreno sold the patent of this device (at the time called radio-film) and with the money thus earned sustained himself until his diploma was re-validated (in 1926) and he could start practising medicine at Mount Sinai Hospital in New York.

Based on his work with the spontaneous theatre and the living newspaper, Moreno realized various radio programmes. He believed that through this means of mass communication he could do psychodrama sessions involving great numbers of people. However, his interest in the potential of radio decreased as he perceived this means of communication turning into a cultural conserve, losing its most important characteristic: spontaneity (live broadcasts were gradually replaced by pre-recorded programmes). Eventually, with the rise of television (at the beginning of the 1940s), Moreno's interest in radio had disappeared completely.

However, before we look at Moreno's psychodramatic experience with television, it is important to first highlight his preceding interest in cinema. Driven by his investigative spirit, he explored the production techniques of film, and presented proposals for therapeutic films to various producers.

In 1933, while working with a group of women at a reformatory in Hudson, Moreno made a 12-minute long silent film entitled 'The training of a waitress'. The film was presented at the assembly of the American Psychiatry Association, in Washington, in May 1935. Even though it does not represent a classical psychodrama session, this film is significant from the perspective of professional training, or *role-playing*. It can be considered as one of the first steps towards our modern action methods, used in organizational psychodrama (action techniques used within companies) for training purposes. We could say that Moreno was also a pioneer within this area.

Moreno's second film was entitled 'Introduction to psychodrama'. It was a coloured talking film, realized in the early 1940s with didactic purposes. In this film Moreno talks about and demonstrates certain aspects of psychodrama, such as the psychodramatic stage and the techniques of self-presentation, role-reversal and double. Later on he realized two more therapeutic films entitled 'Psychodrama, group psychotherapy in action' and 'Marriage psychodrama'.

In 1964 Moreno did a full psychodramatic film at the Camarillo State Hospital (a psychiatric hospital) in California. He arrived there with two teams (a psychodrama team and a camera crew) and filmed a psychodrama (involving patients, doctors and nurses) on the theme of discharge from the hospital. Moreno's objective was to present the film in other hospitals, for other groups of patients, doctors and nurses, using it as a therapeutic film. He believed that the film may help other patients ready to leave hospital gain insights regarding their own discharge, bring to the surface their feelings connected to the discharge and experience catharsis.

In section IX, entitled 'Therapeutic motion pictures' of his book 'Psychodrama' Moreno (1946) describes the method he used for the realization of therapeutic films. He clearly states that a therapeutic film does not simply mean the filming of a psychodrama; what he proposes is a different method, developing in stages. In the first stage, unfolding in various scenes, a protagonist dramatizes the different aspects of his main conflict. Following this, the scenes are further refined in order to compose a script, which is then filmed. Finally, the material is exhibited for a test-audience who will decide which parts of it should be kept for the final script.

Moreno describes three different methods for making therapeutic films. Within the first option the patient himself is the main actor of his drama, appearing in the film as himself, the production of the film being part of his treatment. The patient is 'assisted by a number of auxiliary egos, a type of specialized, therapeutic actor, who portray the complementary roles which the patient needs in the course of the film story' (Moreno 1946, p.395). In the second method the protagonist is represented by an auxiliary ego; the protagonist may also appear in the film in a secondary role, but no-one will know that the material comes from him. In the third possibility, the protagonist participates only in the first stage of dramatizing his scene, but he does not appear on the actual film (even though he is present at the filming). The protagonist only supplies the material dramatized by auxiliary egos (one of them taking on his role). In this way, the private world of the patient is totally protected, assuring the confidentiality of the therapeutic material. In all three methods the main objective is the patient's psychotherapy; the work is done for the protagonist's benefit, while helping the second audience (to whom the film may be exhibited) is only secondary. According to Moreno:

> in therapeutic motion pictures, film or television, the selection of conflicts, the construction of plots, the choice and training of cast, must be made in accord with psychodramatic principles. ...Although the adequate production of a therapeutic film is important, it has to be realized that the main object of a therapeutic motion picture is not the production process but the treatment of audiences. (Moreno 1946, p. 390)

It was in 1942 that Moreno first entered a television studio. Observing the functioning of this mass media vehicle (which at that time only broadcasted live programmes), he wrote a study regarding psychodrama and television. In this he described the way television and the studio worked, and proposed a method for the recording of psychodrama sessions. He believed that through the exhibition of psychodramas on television, millions of people could be reached. He dreamed of breaking down the walls of consultation rooms (to which psychodrama was confined) and reaching 'social reality'. In one of his texts he wrote: 'It is advisable to organize psychodrama sessions that, through the means of a television station, can reach the whole world.' However, Moreno was never able to realize this proposal.

Continuing the path of Moreno

Since 1980 I have been working with a group of people with the intention of recovering and reviving this proposal of Moreno and adapting it to our present times. I believe that Moreno's idea can be accomplished, and that this is one of the possible paths that mass therapy (considered to be a utopian dream in Moreno's day) may follow. Since the time when Moreno made this proposal, technology and the world of communication has gone through a process of development and change, enabling us to use more advanced equipment for the recording of images.

In Brazil, video-recorders started to become popular during the 1980s. However, in the early 1970s I had already had the opportunity to attend a workshop of José Angelo Gaiarsa, who recorded images while working with body language. At that time José Fonseca had also experimented with recording group and couple therapy sessions. From this first contact with filmed footage I started to think about the possibility of uniting video and psychodrama. The idea of recording sessions and then studying them in detail fascinated me.

My first experience in connecting psychodrama to video dates back to 13 April 1980, when I recorded an 8-hour-long marathon group therapy process. Following this, I started to record a monthly session with all four of my ongoing therapy groups. Over a period of 18 months we recorded more than a hundred video-psychodramas that were only presented to the group members and were only used for study purposes. For ethical reasons these films were never exhibited to any other audience.

In May 1980, together with a group of other psychodramatists we recorded a psychodrama session based on the dynamics of the here-and-now; this time our objective was to also exhibit the film to people outside the group (second audience). The Group of Experimental Video-psychodrama (GEV) was formed, a group that continued to work until December 1980. Together with this group we studied various aspects of the video-psychodrama, recording 21 sessions. Based on this research, I wrote a monograph entitled 'Video-psychodrama' (Pamplona da Costa 1980).

In 1981, we were invited by Sulamita Mareines (an artist) to undertake a video-psychodrama session in an art gallery. In Mareines's studio, the group members were interacting with the objects and space, while the session was recorded. Some time later we did another psychodrama together with Mareines at the São Paulo Museum of Image and Sound, following the presentation of her 'Theatre of objects' (an exhibition of talking sculptures). Later on, we recorded numerous other video-psychodramas with various groups at symposiums and conferences.

Invited by Regina Monteiro, in April 1984 (at the end of the military regime) we did a video-psychodrama at the São Paulo City Hall entitled 'The psychodrama of free elections'. I co-directed the session with Regina and

Carlos Borba was recording. In 1984, at a video festival organized at the São Paulo Museum of Image and Sound, we did a 'psychodrama without words' with the group of musician psychodramatists; the group was improvising music together with the singer Rosa Maria.

In August 1985, we produced 'The psychodrama of AIDS' at the São Paulo City Hall, which was followed by a debate on the topic. In September, as the closing act of the First Symposium of Men we presented the 'Psychodrama of men'; this work formed the basis of the book entitled 'Macho, masculinity, man' (Pamplona da Costa 1986).

In May 1989, the first street video-psychodrama was recorded, working with the theme of mental asylums. The session (sponsored by the Health Department of the City of São Paulo) was co-directed by me and Regina Monteiro and recorded by Carlos Borba. Two years later Regina Monteiro and Vania Crelier directed two more street sessions that were also recorded.

The above repeatedly-mentioned term of 'video-psychodrama' was formulated by me to denominate the working method of recording psychodrama sessions onto video, with the ultimate objective of exhibiting them on closed circuit television (CCTV). Video-psychodrama was also the first step in the direction of my work with tele-psychodrama (exhibiting recorded psychodrama sessions on open television). So, before presenting my studies and experiences with tele-psychodrama, first I will describe some aspects and possible applications of video-psychodrama.

The use of video-psychodrama in therapy sessions

As I mentioned previously, in 1980 I was recording one monthly session with my four ongoing therapy groups. The material thus produced was used to deepen and refine the work and experience of the group members. When recording such therapy sessions, the exhibition of the recorded material is limited only to the group itself (first audience); there is no possibility for exhibiting this work to another person or group (second audience). The only exception to this rule is the presentation of the material to a supervisor (if the group agrees to this).

Video-psychodrama sessions are recorded by another psychodramatist, whom I call 'video-director', that is, video-psychodrama is the video-director's view of the session. It is important that the video-director is also a psychodramatist, who knows and is familiar with the psychodrama method. Since the video-director is part of the therapeutic team, his role as a psychotherapist, should be well developed. A video or television technician (not trained in psychodrama) would not have sufficient knowledge of how to record a therapeutic session and so would not be able to produce a video-psychodrama.

Beyond the social, group and dramatic context (characteristic to psychodrama), video-psychodrama is also characterized by a 'video-psychodramatic context' which consists of the video equipment and the video-director. Even though this latter does not participate verbally, he 'interferes' with the group and the dramatic context.

Psychodrama has five basic elements: the stage, the protagonist, the director, the auxiliary ego and the audience. In video-psychodrama we need to consider at least one more element: the video-director with the video equipment. If we need to use a second camera for the recording, we will need one more element, the so-called 'psycho-cameraman'. Some alterations of the five basic elements may also be necessary:

- The *stage* for example, should be clearly delimited. It should consist of a space that allows the video-director to move around without difficulty, in order to obtain the best view of the dramatic scene. To keep the audience (of the dramatic action) involved, scenes should be directed towards them, with the objective of achieving a resonance with the protagonist. We will need to do the same in relation to the video-director and his camera in case it is not possible for him (or her) to move around easily.

- It is also important that the *protagonist* is comfortable with and used to being filmed. In my experience this soon happens after a few sessions of recording. Groups assimilate the camera very well, and after a while 'forget' about its presence.

- Beyond his usual functions, the *director* also needs to have a good connection with the video-director. During therapy sessions the director has a specific role: he needs to be attentive towards and give instructions for the video-director. For example, he may instruct the video-director in a loud voice: 'Come closer and see what is going on here', or, in a lowered voice: 'Try to film so and so from that angle.' The video-director however, does not talk during the session (since he is close to the microphone, his voice would interfere with the recording). The director should also always remember that (due to his handling of the camera) the video-director may have a different view from his own.

- *The auxiliary ego* also needs to be attentive to the signals and instructions of the director. Through his function as an actor, he needs to contribute to the action in such a way that during the later exhibition of the video, it becomes explicit what happened during the dramatic action. As part of his function of social observer, he can elicit things that happen to the protagonist and which will facilitate the work of the director and video-director.

- *Group members* who are not taking part in the dramatic action are also recorded by the camera; they are the audience. Part of the video-director's skill is to be able to also film the audience without losing the focus of the dramatic action.

- I would also like to include here some thoughts regarding the *video-director*, as an extra element of video-psychodrama. I have already mentioned that the video-director should be a psychodramatist; however, he also needs to have some basic knowledge and skill regarding the use of the video equipment. It is important to clarify that the video-director is not an auxiliary ego.

- In therapy groups, where the work is centred on the protagonist, the video-director will only focus on this group (without considering a second audience). The psychodramatic director will also have as a priority his relationship to the video-director while the technical conditions for a good recording (lights, proximity of the camera, etc.) will become secondary issues.

- As a therapist himself, the video-director may experience moments of distress. At times, the content of the recorded scenes may generate deep feelings in him. The video-director needs to be able to contain these feelings during the recording and express them only in the exhibition stage of the video-psychodrama, when he can share with the group.

- It can also happen that an individual protagonist doesn't want a certain issue to be recorded. The protagonist may even not want the video-director to be present. As the recording is considered a means of the therapeutic work, we need to respect the protagonist's wish and cannot impose the use of this instrument; however, it is important to clarify why the protagonist does not want the recording, this may enlighten certain hidden aspects of his/her issue.

- In order to have a good flow in the work, it is necessary for the video-director to have a good relationship with the patients. This means that it may even be necessary to allow the dramatization of this relationship (video–director/patients) in order to overcome possible difficulties within it. Generally speaking, groups and clients respond well to the recording of their sessions when they understand the benefits resulting from this. Video-psychodrama should be only applied if this is for the benefit of the client(s).

Beyond the warm-up, dramatization and sharing, a therapeutic video-psychodrama session also has an *exhibition* phase. This may be followed by further phases, such as *processing* and *supervision*.

Since the phases of the warm-up, dramatization and sharing are well known to all psychodramatists, I will not discuss them in detail. Let us look instead at the *exhibition* phase. Within this phase, all members of the therapeutic team as well as the clients have the same role, that of the viewer or spectator. It is also obvious however, that nobody disposes of their previous role. Thus, we have: director–viewer, auxiliary ego–viewer, video-director–viewer and client–viewer. In a sense, this phase allows a greater horizontality of roles. Everybody observes him/herself and the others, and vice-versa. It can be a very rich experience for all, because the patients can see themselves in action while the therapeutic team can clarify certain aspects of the session.

The exhibition of the recorded session can foster insights and catharsis, resulting in deep emotional experiences for the clients. However, the director, auxiliary ego and video-director can also benefit from the comments of the clients (for example, 'What you did at that moment helped me', or 'What you did at that moment wasn't useful') regarding their performance in these roles. Recordings may be replayed many times, at normal speed, in slow motion, or frame by frame, with the objective of facilitating the elaboration of the session (with the participation of all); video-psychodrama can also serve as a kind of feed-back by the patients regarding the therapeutic roles.

We talk about the phase of *processing* when only the therapists try to gain an understanding of the process from a theoretical and technical point of view. If, for example, we work with a didactic group, that is, with students who seek to learn by experiencing psychodrama, the video-psychodrama can be exhibited twice: the first time with a therapeutic purpose (elaboration), and the second time with a didactic purpose or processing, with the participation of all group members.

The next phase of video-psychodrama – that is, *supervision* with a supervisor therapist – depends completely on the approval and permission of the patients. Issues of confidentiality and professional ethics play an important role here. When taking a psychodrama session to supervision, what we study is the internalized session, from which we leave out personal information in order to avoid the identification of the involved persons. In the case of video-psychodrama however, it is impossible to prevent the identification of the people and clients, because they are recorded on video. Since the sociometric network of therapist and clients is strongly interwoven, I suggest letting the group know which professional will do the supervision. The consent of the group should be only asked after they have seen the film of their session, and this should be recorded on video or in writing.

We also need to distinguish the stages in the making of a video-psychodrama. These are:

- *The production stage* – this is the recording stage, or the group moment. There are certain aspects or variables that need to be taken into consideration at this stage. For example, a television set can be used at the same time with the recording, allowing the instant viewing of the recorded images. Another variable is the video-camera, generally considered as an instrument that gives 'therapeutic objectivity'; however, strictly speaking, it cannot be used as an intermediary object.[2] And finally the variable of lights, which should be more intense when making a colour recording.

- *The stage of editing or montage* – this is the stage of choosing which images to include or cut from the film. It can be done by the therapists only, or by the group itself. If the editing is done with the whole group, this stage coincides with the following (exhibition).

- *The exhibition stage* – this is the stage when the patients and therapists view the recorded video-psychodrama, trying to extract from it all the elements necessary for psychotherapy. This stage is necessary and it should be accomplished during the actual session with enough time allocated for it. As mentioned above, the video-psychodrama may be exhibited to a second audience consisting of one or more supervisors (supervision phase), this being a phase for therapists only.

In the following I will present some other possibilities for using video-psychodrama with therapeutic purposes.

Individual psychodrama with video-psychodrama

When working with an individual client, we also invite and work together with a video-director. The session follows the same phases as when working with a group (these phases were presented above), using the same video-psychodrama contexts and elements.

Another possibility in individual work is for the director to also assume the role of the video-director. The director would place the camera at a reasonable distance, turning it in the direction of the protagonist when he/she takes on different roles, using the zoom when necessary. With a bit of creativity, the director can create further possibilities of using video-psychodrama in one-to-one sessions.

Using video-psychodrama in couple or family psychodrama

For these applications, an auxiliary ego and a video-director are also present. Since the protagonist is a couple or a family, and (beyond the three members of the therapeutic team) there are no other clients present, the video-psychodrama is assumed with more importance. Elaboration becomes more profound, because the sharing only involves the clients and the therapists. The recorded images will greatly facilitate the perception of each person involved.

However, considering our economic situation in Brazil, using more than one psychotherapist in a therapeutic session is a bit of a luxury; most of the time we work without an auxiliary ego and without a video-director. It is more realistic to use video-psychodrama within training organizations (universities, or psychodrama institutes and societies), inviting a psychodrama student to be the video-director, since he is more interested in learning than in the financial benefit.

Using a therapeutic video as a warm-up for a therapeutic group

We experimented with showing only parts of a recorded video-psychodrama, stopping the exhibition when the conflict becomes clear, but before the resolution is reached. Using this as a warm-up, we continue to work with the group, who through their identification with the characters presented on the video, are asked to find a solution for that particular situation.

Video-psychodrama and closed circuit television (CCTV)

Video recorders and players can be easily connected in a circuit, thus transmitting recorded images. Such a circuit can be used when we cannot bring all participants together within the same room. We could have, for example, 30 people in the room where the video-psychodrama happens (with the participation of the director, video-director and auxiliary ego), while the recorded images are instantly transmitted to another five locations, with 50 people in each. So, altogether there are 280 people involved. Each group watching the transmitted images of the video-psychodrama is facilitated by a psychodramatist who, after the exhibition, invites the group to share and elaborate. This modality can be used in schools, psychiatric hospitals, prisons, or even psychodrama conferences, allowing the therapist to direct without the discomfort of an over-crowded room.

Another objective for the use of CCTV is to investigate how video-psychodrama is received when presented only through television. Moreno suggested the presentation of therapeutic films on CCTV, that is, exhibiting video-psychodramas to a second audience (in either one or more other locations). In such a situation the audience should be warmed up for the exhibition and later on their responses and reactions should be observed. (It differs from what I call tele-psychodrama, made to be exhibited on open television. This working modality will be presented in the next section.)

This is the exhibition phase when the video-psychodrama reaches an audience of people or professionals who did not take part in the actual making of the film. This second audience may vary depending on the purpose and the size of the group to whom the film was destined. The second audience can consist of a small group (exhibition with a normal television), a bigger group (big screen) or masses (presentation through channels).

The second audience should be warmed up for the exhibition. It is also important to create an appropriate climate for the exhibition. The room should be darkened, quiet and relaxed. The director will ask the audience members to relax in order to receive the scenes of the video-psychodrama and to reflect on their emotions provoked by them.

As I mentioned above, in the 1980s, after a year and a half of working with therapy groups as well as individual clients, we started to record public psychodrama and sociodrama sessions. The fact that these sessions were public already implied that they could be recorded and exhibited to other groups of spectators, but even so, we still clearly explained to the participants of these public sessions why we were recording and what our objective was: to present the material in other open sessions aiming to unchain new views on the themes that were addressed, or to lead into new sessions. As seen above, most of these experiences were focused on social issues, such as free elections, urban violence or AIDS.

I would like to present here another of our experiences from the 1980s: the recording and exhibition of a therapeutic video-psychodrama.

This was a unique experience with the participation of Regina Dourado, a television actress. She had never participated in a psychotherapy session before and she did not know us; nevertheless she accepted our invitation to participate in the recording of a therapeutic act. We worked with emotional issues presented by her, letting her decide at the end if the footage could be exhibited publicly or not.

The session lasted for three hours and the participants consisted of Regina, two auxiliary egos, the video-director and myself as director.

Our original agreement was that Regina would only provide the material for the story, and that her participation in the filmed scene would be limited to a secondary role. But, as the session moved on, she got involved and entered the role of the protagonist with such power that I felt it would be wrong to stop her. I gave up our original plan and directed her – she became the main actress of her own drama.

The three-hour long session was edited and reduced into a 50-minute film that, with Regina's authorization, was presented at scientific meetings, conferences, seminars and lectures (second audiences). Later on, the film was further reduced to 40 minutes.

During these exhibitions I always learnt something new regarding how to achieve better results. I developed a proper warm-up technique: I try to achieve an atmosphere similar to that of a cinema. When placing a television in front of people, we can observe that the role of television spectator is so natural and developed in them, that they will act as they would be at home (where they wake up, go to the kitchen, the bathroom, talk on the phone, eat popcorn and converse). I try to avoid this happening. I prepare people for a cinema atmosphere. I close the doors and ask them not to talk. I want the spectator to be immersed in Regina's world.

This film can be used in different ways. It can serve as an example of psychodrama for psychodrama trainees (discussing the techniques used by the director; or the work of the auxiliary egos), and it can also be a useful instrument for a therapy session for the people who are watching it.

However, both of the above foci demand a different kind of warm-up of the spectators. When exhibiting the film for psychodrama trainees, I ask them to make their observations based on their trainee role, looking at the work of the director and the auxiliaries. If working in a therapy group, before exhibiting the film I call the members' attention to Reginas's issues; I want them to be open and let Regina's world enter them and mix with their own.

The results of this work are generally very positive and they confirm Moreno's proposal. The participants' (second audience) degree of identification is high, and generally leads to some people getting emotional, crying, having insights and arriving at catharsis. The exhibition of the film is followed by the phase of sharing, giving a chance for everybody to say what the protagonist awoke in them. Generally, this is sufficient to round up the emotions of that encounter (which usually lasts for two hours). However, at times, a short vignette is necessary to finalize issues for the spectators.

The advantage of such a video footage is that it can be reproduced. Imagine a footage dealing with the theme of discharge from mental health hospitals – the issue also treated by Moreno. It is possible to make hundreds of copies of it, distribute them to medical or psychological institutions working with this client group, and see what results it would bring. I believe that, because it originates in the theatre, psychodrama is the only psychotherapeutic trend that has this potential. If we would try to exhibit a film of a verbal psychotherapy session, spectators would probably lose interest after a few minutes. All forms of exclusively verbal psychotherapies are unviable when presented publicly. The reason for this is clear: psychodrama takes the patient for a journey inside him/herself, transforming his experiences through psychodramatic scenes. It is done through dramatic action – it is this aspect within which the great potential of television and cinema lies.

Tele-psychodrama – psychodrama on open television

As a result of around 400 hours of video-recordings, in 1984 I wrote an article entitled 'Tele-psychodrama', in which I proposed the making of a pilot psychodrama project on open television. Within this article I described the various possibilities of using psychodrama in television, I presented issues that may awake the interest of the public, and even gave methodological details for the production of such programmes. This text however, remains unpublished to this day, maybe because it described a proposal too advanced for the time. After all, Brazilian television was very different in 1984. At the time there were no programmes that would have an interest in the public exhibition of the private lives of people. This however, radically changed in the 1990s, with the appearance of a stunning invasion of private life, and with the electronic media exposing without selection scenes of war, homicide, suicide and human degradation – a change that in my view has a very strong counter-educational potential. People appear on television ready to strip to their most intimate emotions, in front of an audience more and more eager for this kind of personal and private disclosure.

In the 1980s however, I was told that exposing people on television was a crazy idea, and that my proposal (or rather Moreno's proposal) seemed to be utopian. (Just imagine what people thought about Moreno in the discrete decade of the 1940s – they must have thought he was out of his mind!) In 1993, together with Carlos Borba, we were invited by Heloísa Dupas Penteado (a sociologist and educator, and an enthusiast for psychodrama) to do pedagogical video-psychodramas with the students of the Educational Section of the São Paulo University. The outcome of these recordings was excellent and we resumed this experience of pedagogical video-psychodrama within a research agenda of pedagogical tele-psychodrama. The idea and proposal for this research once again came from Heloísa Penteado at the end of 1999.

This project involved a multidisciplinary team of psychodrama, education, communication and television professionals and it was denominated 'Pedagogical tele-psychodrama, education and the pedagogy of communication'. What the project proposed was the connection of two languages: the languages of television and psychodrama. The first part of the project consisted in the encounter between psychodrama techniques and television techniques in order to create tele-psychodrama. The second step involved the exhibition of the recorded tele-psychodramas in schools (on closed circuit television) and educational television channels (open circuit television); the exhibition was followed by the questioning of television spectators regarding the educational effectiveness of the programme.

The first step of the project (that is the production of the tele-psychodrama) in itself already implied an educative process. The relationship between the researching psychodramatists, teachers, students and other employees of the school was in accordance with the theoretical-practical postulates of pedagogical psychodrama. It was a hard and taxing task, but also joyful. This was our overriding impression all through the year 2000 while working within the school, in the administrative, pedagogical and psychodrama meetings, during the production of tele-psychodramas, the preparation, as well as during the exhibition phases of the video.

All this work was done on a voluntary basis, without any financial sponsorship, and therefore without the possibility of recording in a real television studio. We worked with domestic video cameras, and without appropriate conditions of space, light, sound, etc.

It was in 2001 that we finally had the chance to improve on these technical difficulties thanks to a partnership with the post-graduate programme of the Casper Líbero Social Communication School. This partnership was made possible by Liana Gotlieb (psychodrama pedagogue), who became part of the research co-ordination team, and enabled us to record tele-psychodrama sessions in a television studio.

Once again, I became hopeful that my proposal for making tele-psychodramas adequate for exhibition on open television may turn into reality. I strongly believe that tele-psychodrama would have immense possibilities within a television network. However, the directors of television channels are still reluctant to see this, and it is difficult to convince them.

The great challenge

After having seen spectators' reactions to Regina's psychodrama (these were CCTV exhibitions), I started to think how such presentations would work on open television, and what reactions they would unchain in the television spectators. One of my main concerns was that the home atmosphere of the television spectator is different from that of audiences specially prepared (warmed-up) for this kind of exhibition. As I mentioned above, the role of the television spectator is natural to most people, and is connected to an environment where he/she (the spectator) eats popcorn, listens to the dog barking, argues with family members – and perhaps therefore wouldn't get involved in the drama presented on the television (or, may even think that it is just a fictitious story).

So my main preoccupation concerned language. What we use in psychotherapeutic video-psychodrama exhibited on CCTV and under special conditions that facilitate the spectators' concentration, cannot be the same in the case of tele-psychodrama exhibited on open television. Since I cannot ask the television spectators to disconnect the telephone, to forget about the fridge, the dog and the neighbours, I would need to produce something that is capable of involving them despite domestic distractions, something that can provoke and capture their attention.

My great challenge was how to create this new, tele-psychodramatic language, as a union of the already developed video-graphic and psychodramatic languages. This demanded a refinement, not just from a technical perspective (aiming at attracting the attention of the television spectator and obtain his involvement), but also from a psychodramatic point of view (in the sense of selecting the 'best scenes', which are most appropriate for the possible unfolding of understanding). This demanded cuts and the re-editing of the filmed footages, as well as a situation where it is easy and possible for both recording technicians and psychodramatists to work together. I have the privilege of working together with a very experienced video-director (Carlos Borba) who, beyond being a psychodramatist, also has some experience with theatre and cinematography. Thus, he has a special eye for detecting and filming the most tense aspects of a certain scene, producing footages that fulfil the demands of this new, tele-psychodramatic language.

The second great challenge regarding the presentation of video-psychodrama on open television networks was the technique. These films need to have excellent quality of image and sound, a quality much better than that of video-psychodramas produced only for exhibition on closed circuit. This presupposes the use of a proper television studio with three or four cameras, good microphones, an adequate lighting system and a well delimited psychodramatic space providing good visibility for the television spectator.

Another question concerns the people participating in the psychodrama. There are an infinite number of themes and issues of community interest that could be addressed on television (such as the readjustment of convicts, life in the slums, child adoption, etc.), and in the case of each one we need to consider the presence of people who are directly involved and related to these issues.

The work within the television studio can also involve people who are not taking part directly in the psychodrama session. If working with ten people in a scene, I will usually have another 30 people assisting (watching). This audience represents the television spectator, and although they are more distanced than those who are in the scene, I will still need to pay attention to them and to take into consideration their responses, because they will help in the final editing of the programme.

In order to achieve a good degree of involvement of this studio audience, they need to be adequately warmed-up; this is done by a second psychodramatist, acting as the director of the audience (he will not be seen by the television spectators, and his work starts before the recording of the programme). He prepares and warms up the audience, making them ready to participate in the recording, taking in consideration the specific characteristics of this work (it is not a common show to be watched, but something that will be born spontaneously during the action). The warm-up of the audience should also be recorded. Interesting, creative, touching or involving situations often arise within this phase, that would be lost if not recorded.

Ideally there should be plenty of time for the recording. After the adequate preparation of the audience, the actual session and its recording requires around an hour-and-a-half to two hours. This is followed by the editing of the recorded material (reducing it to about 20 to 30 minutes).

After the editing, the director also needs to record certain insertions for the filmed footage. At the opening of the tele-psychodrama he addresses the television spectator, explaining what is going to happen, talking about psychodrama and the chosen theme. Further to this, he also appears during the presentation of the programme, making comments and offering further explanations. At the end he also needs to do a closure, commenting on the resolution that has been reached and making suggestions for the television spectator. He can say for example: 'Maria dramatized her difficulty of saying *no*, and she found "such-and-such" a way to deal with this situation. You, in front of the television may find your own way. Think how you could say *no* to people.' The director opens the possibility and allows for each spectator to find a new response to an old question.

I have no doubts that when presenting this kind of work on television, we (director, auxiliary egos and the members of the group) are running all the risks inherent in such an exhibition. After all, we show something with which nobody had experimented until now (and so there is no set way of doing it correctly), a work that needs to be invented, done and redone until we arrive at an adequate result.

Living according to the principles of psychodrama, however, involves creation, spontaneity, research and the search of new answers to old questions. Risk is inherent in the psychodramatic action.

Conclusions

I believe that considering Moreno's proposals regarding cinema, therapeutic films and television as a starting point, it is possible to produce therapeutic, pedagogical or social video-psychodramas and tele-psychodramas. This is maybe the first step towards sociatry, which is considered by many psychodramatists to be a Morenian utopia. It is the search for the limits of our possibilities, a search for how far psychodrama can go in being a tool for individual and social transformation.

At the turn of the millennium we have broadband internet that makes the transmission of great numbers of data easier. This will allow for the participants, individuals and groups, to see each other when they talk. We will have then to think about web-psychodrama, a kind of psychodrama that... But this is for another chapter.

Notes

1 This chapter is based on the following two papers: 'Videopsicodrama'. In R.F. Monteiro *Técnicas Fundamentais do Psicodrama [Fundamental Techniques in Psychodrama]*. São Paulo: Ágora, 1993, pp.132–150 and 'Telepsicodrama: um sonho de Moreno em pesquisa'. In R. Pamplona da Costa, R. *Um Homen à Frente de seu Tempo – O Psicodrama de Moreno no Século XXI (A Man Ahead of his Time – Moreno's Psychodrama in the 21st Century)*. São Paulo: Ágora, 2001, pp.189–204.

2 For Bermudez's criteria regarding the intermediary object, see Chapter 5.

Appendix
Directory of the psychodrama organizations affiliated to the Brazilian Psychodrama Federation (FEBRAP)

FEBRAP Federação Brasileiro de Psicodrama (Brazilian Psychodrama Federation)
Rua Cardoso de Almeida 23, Cj.63, Perdizes, 05013-000 São Paulo
www.febrap.org.br info@febrap.org.br

São Paulo Region
ABPS Associação Brasileira de Psicodrama e Sociodrama
Rua Eça de Queiroz 220, Paraiso, 04011-031 São Paulo
www.abps.com.br abps@abps.com.br

ACTO Desenvolvimento Profissional e Pessoal
Rua General Vitorino Monteiro 158, Vila Romana, 05053-060 São Paulo
acto@uol.com.br

ANIMUS Psicodrama e Educação
Rua Cabedelo 365, Morumbi, 05618-010 São Paulo
leilanimus@aol.com

CELEIRO Espaço Sociodramático
Rua Virginio Pereira 1625, Higienópolis, 14405-092 São Paulo
celeiro@francanet.com.br

CICLO de Mutação Cibernética Psicodrama e Psicoterapia
Rua Generosa Bastos 3443, Redentora, 15015-790 São José do Rio Preto
www.ciclomuta.com.br ciclo@ciclomuta.com.br

COSMOS Guarulhos Núcleo de Estudos do Desenvolvimento Pessoal
Rua Francisco Antonio de Miranda 88, 07090-140, Guarulhos-SP
www.institutocosmos.com.br cosmos@institutocosmos.com.br

COSMOS Campinas Instituto Cosmos de Campinas
Rua Barbosa da Cunha 887, Jd. Guanabara, 13073-320 Campinas-SP
cosmocamp@hotmail.com

EMC Equilibrio, Mente e Corpo Consultoria
Rua Purpurina 131, Cj.76, Vila Madalena, 05435-030 São Paulo
celinasob@uol.com.br

EPP Escola Paulista de Psicodrama
Rua Cel. Artur de Paula Ferreira 28, Vila Nova Conceição, 04511-060 São Paulo
www.epp.psc.br epp@epp.psc.br

EPS Escola de Psicodrama de Sorocaba
Rua Antonio José Castro Novo 345, 18095-070 Sorocaba-SP
psicodramasorocaba@hotmail.com

F&Z Assessoria e Desenvolvimento em Educação e Saúde
Rua Jose Jamarelli 199, Cj.96, Morumbi, 05615-001 São Paulo
www.terapiafamiliar.med.br p.za@terra.com.br

GETEP Grupo de Estudos de Técnicas Psicodramáticas
Rua Dr. Paulo Vieria 17, Sumare, 01257-000 São Paulo
getep@terra.com.br

IBAP Instituto Bauruense de Psicodrama
Rua Rafael Mercadante 2-59, Jd. Estoril, 17045-130 Bauru-SP
www.ibaponline.hpg.com.br ibaponline@ieg.com.br

IPPGC Instituto de Psicodrama e Psicoterapia de Grupo de Campinas
Rua Angelino Rossi 12, Jd. Botafogo, 13070-231 Campinas-SP
ippgc@terra.com.br

IPRP Instituto de Psicodrama de Ribeirão Preto
Rua Altino Arantes 1774, Jd. América, 14020-200 Ribeirão Preto-SP
iprp-owner@yahoogrupos.com.br

IPR Instituto de Politicas Relacionais
Rua Araujo 124, 3255-9570 São Paulo
relacionais@relacionais.org.br

IRP Instituto Rio Pretense de Psicodrama
Rua São Paulo 1606, 15060-035 São José de Rio Preto-SP
i.r.p.@terra.com.br

POTENCIAR Consultores Associados
Rua Felix Braguemond 26, Pinheiros, 05427-040 São Paulo
www.potenciar.com.br potenciar@potenciar.co.br

SEDES Depto Psicodrama Instituto Sedes Sapientae
Rua Ministro Godoy 1484, Perdizes, 05015-900 São Paulo
www.sedes.org.br psicodrama@sedes.org.br

SOPSP Sociedade de Psicodrama de São Paulo
Rua Dos Ingleses 74, Bela Vista, 01329-000 São Paulo
www.sopsp.org.br sopsp@uol.com.br

SOSAP Sociedade Santista de Psicodrama
Rua Barão de Paranapiacaba 16, 11050-250 Santos-SP
carias@iron.com.br

SOVAP Sociedade Paulistana de Psicodrama
Rua Pamplona 33, Casa 2, Bela Vista, 01405-030 São Paulo

South Region

IDH Instituto de Desenvolvimento Humano
Av. Itaqui 174, Petropolis, 90460-140 Porto Alegre-RS
www.idhumano.com.br idhumano@idhumano.com.br

CONTEXTO Associação de Psicodrama do Paraná
Rua Desembergador Motta 2898, Centro, 80430-200 Curitiba-PR
www.contexto.com.br aldojunior@onda.com.br

COSMOS Instituto Cosmos de Joinville
Rua Blumenau 178, 89204-250 Joinville-SC
mbboebel@acquaplant.com.br

PARTNER RH Consultoria Desenvolvimento e Prestação de Serviços
Av. Hoton Gama D'Eça 900, 88015-240 Florianóplis-SC
locuspartner@msn.com

ATUARE Sociedade de Psicodrama Atuare
Rua Esteves Junior 366, 88010-000 Florianopolis-SC
atuare@intercorp.com.br

SPP Sociedade Paranaense de Psicodrama
Av. Mar. Floriano Peixoto 2490, Rebouças, 80220-000 Curitiba-PR
spp30anos@teraa.com.br

North-Northeast Region

ASBAP Associação Bahiana de Psicodrama e Psicoterapia de Grupo
Rua Itatuba 201, 40275-350 Salvador-BA
asbap@uol.com.br

CEPS Centro de Psicodrama e Sociodrama
Av. Euclides da Cunha 475, ap.601, 40150-120 Salvador-BA
ceps.ba@uol.com.br

FEPS Fundação de Estudos e Pesquisas Socionômicas do Brasil
Av. Antonio Sales 1885, 60135-101 Fortaleza-CE
wedja@fepsdobrasil.org.br

Instituto de Psicodrama e Mascaras de Fortaleza
Av. Senador Virgilio Tavora 867, Casa 75, Aldeota, 60170-250 Fortaleza-CE
marcoamato@terra.com.br

COSMOS Instituto Cosmos de Recife
Rua das Pernambucanas 407, Graças, 52011-010 Recife-PE
cristenorio@bol.com.br

PROFINT Profissionais Integrados
Praça da Bandeira 465, 49010-470 Aracaju-Sergipe
profint@sergipenet.com.br

MATRIZ CRIATIVA Núcleo de Ação e Desenvolvimento
Rua Cravalho Lima 38, Aldeota, 60125-040 Fortaleza-CE
matrizcriativa@fortalnet.com.br

SOPSBA Sociedade de Psicodrama da Bahia
Av. Tancredo Neves 1189, 41080-021 Salvador-BA
www.sopsba.org.br sopsba@sopsba.org.br

Mid-West Region

ABP Associação Brasiliense de Psicodrama e Sociodrama
SCRS, 514 - Bloco B - sl. 1/5, 70380-525 Brasília-DF
abp.ibp@ig.com.br

CENAS Csa das Cenas - O Psicodrama Mineiro
Rua Javari 383, Osório, 38400-146 Uberlândia-MG
cassildaborges@mg.dilk.com.br

CEPB Centro de Psicodrama de Brasília
SGAS 910, Cj.B, Bl.D, sl.227, 70390-100 Brasília-DF
mmarra@terra.com.br

CPP Clínica de Psicologia e Psicodrama
SCN Q2 Lote Director Bl.A sl.407, 70310-500 Brasília-DF
cppdf@terra.com.br

FOCUS Consultoria em Relacionamentos Interpessoais
SHIG/Sul Qda 706 Bl.C, casa 03, Asa Sul, 70350-753 Brasília-DF
focus@solar.com.br

GAYA Instituto Gaya de Psicodrama
Rua Frederico Komdofer 117, Jd. Dos Estados, 79020-270 Campo Grande-MS
gaya@gaya.com.br

SOGEP Sociedade Goiana de Psicodrama
Rua Sete 165, Setor Aeroporto, 74075-230 Goiânia-GO
sogep@netgo.com.br

South-East Region

DELPHOS Delphos Espaço Psico-Social
Rua João Afonso 20, Humaita, 22261-040 Rio de Janeiro-RJ
www.delphospsic.com.br delphospsic@uol.com.br

IMPSI Instituto Mineiro de Psicodrama Jacob Levi Moreno
Rua Rio Grande de Norte 1289, sl.501/502, Savassi, 30130-131 Belo Horizonte-MG
impsi@hotmail.com

PEGASUS Pegasus Desenvolvimento e Consultoria
Rua João Galerante 130, Jucutuquara, 29042-110 Vitória-ES
www.pegasusdesenvolvimento.com.br pegasusd@terra.com.br

SOBRAP Soc. Brasileira de Psic. Dinamica e Psicodrama - Regional Juiz de For a
Rua Oswaldo Cruz 198, Santa Helena, 36015-430 Juiz de For a-MG
sobrap@acessa.com

SOMOPSI Sociedade Moreniana de Psicodrama
Rua Haddock Lobo 369, sl.805, Tijuca, 20260-131 Rio de Janeiro-RJ
somopsi@zipmail.com.br

References

Aguiar, M. (1988) *Teatro da Anarquia: um Resgate do Psicodrama (The Theatre of Anarchy: Rescuing Psychodrama)*. Campinas: Papirus.

Aguiar, M. (1991) *A evolução dos conceitos tele e transferência (The evolution of the concepts of tele and transference)*. Round table discussion at the fourth International Psychodrama Encounter, São Paulo.

Aguinis, M. (1996) *Elogio de la Culpa (Praise for the Guilt)*. Buenos Aires: Planet.

Aguinis, M. (1999) *Los Iluminados (The Enlightened)*. Buenos Aires: Atlántida.

Almeida, W.C. (1982) *Psicoterapia Aberta: o Método do Psicodrama (Open Psychotherapy: The Psychodrama Method)*. São Paulo: Agora.

Altenfelder, L. (2001) *Psicoterapia de Grupo com Psicóticos (Group Psychotherapy with Psychotics)*. São Paulo: Lemos Editorial.

American Psychiatric Association (1995) *Manual de Diagnóstico e Estatístico de Transtornos Mentais (Diagnostic and Statistical Manual of Mental Disorders)*. Fourth Edition, Porto Alegre: Artes Médicas.

Angelo, C. (1995) 'A escolha do parceiro' (Choosing a partner). In M. Andolfi, C. Angelo and C. Saccu *O Casal em Crise (The Couple in Crisis)*. São Paulo: Summus.

Berenstein, I. (1990) *Psicoanalisar una Familia (Psychoanalysis of a Family)*. Buenos Aires: Paidós.

Blatner, H. (1969/1970) 'Commentaires sur quelques réserves ordinairement faites concernant le pychodrame.' *Bull. Psychol.*, 23, pp.957–960.

Bowen, M. (1978) *Family Therapy in Clinical practise*. New York: Jason Aronson.

Buarque de Holanda, A.F. (1975) *Novo Dicionário da Lingua Portuguesa (New Portuguese Dictionary)*. São Paulo: Nova Fronteira. Bustos, D.M. *(1974) El Psicodrama (Psychodrama)*. Buenos Aires: Plus Ultra.

Bustos, D.M. (1975) *Psicoterapia Psicodramática (Psychodrama Psychotherapy)*. Buenos Aires: Paidós.

Bustos, D.M. (1979) *O Teste Sociométrico (The Sociometric Test)*. São Paulo: Brasiliense.

Bustos, D.M. (1990) *Perigo... Amor À Vista! (Danger... Love at Sight!)*. São Paulo: Aleph.

Bustos, D.M. (1992) *Freedom, Rehearsals*. São Paulo: Aleph.

Bustos, D.M. (1994) 'Locus, matrix, status nascendi and the concept of clusters.' In P. Holmes, M. Karp and M. Watson *Psychodrama since Moreno*. London and New York: Routledge.

Campedelli, A.M. (1978) 'A propósito do psicodrama bipessoal' (A proposal for bi-personal psychodrama). Dissertation presented at the São Paulo Psychodrama Society.

Coimbra, C. (1995) *Guardiães da Ordem – Uma Viagem pelas Práticas Psi do Brasil do Milagre (The Guardians of Order – A Journey through the Psi practise in Brazil of the Miracles)*. Rio de Janeiro: Oficina do autor.

Cukier, R. (1995) 'Como sobrevivem emocionalmente os seres humanos?' (How do human beings survive emotionally?). *Revista Brasileira de Psicodrama* 3, 2.

D'Andrea, F.F. (1985) Memorial para concurso de professor titular de Psiquiatria FMRP (Memorandum written to obtain the post of Psychiatrist at FMRP). Title obtained in 1985.

Dolto, F. (1992) *Quando os Pais se Separam (When the Parents Separate)*. Rio de Janeiro: Editora Jorge Zahar.

Eco, U. (1991) *Obra Aberta (The Open Composition)*. São Paulo: Perspectiva.

Erikson, E. (1968) *Identidade, Juventude e Crise (Identity, Youth and Crisis)*. Rio de Janeio: Zahar.

Eva, A.C. (1978) 'Grupos terapêuticos psicodramáticos: uma tentetiva de sistematização' (Therapeutic psychodrama groups: an attempt for systematization). *Revista Psicodrama* II, 2, 27–38.

Falivene Alves, L.R. (1990) 'O protagonista: conceito e articulação na teoria e na prática' (The protagonist: the concept and its articulations in the theory and practise). Paper presented at the seventh Brazilian Psychodrama Conference, Rio de Janiero, 1990.

Falivene Alves, L. (1995) 'Jogo: imaginário autorizado e exteriorizado' (Play: authorized and externalized imagination). In J. Mota *O jogo no Psicodrama (Psychodrama and Play)*. São Paulo: Ágora.

Fanchette, J. (1986) *Psicodrama y Teatro Moderno (Psychodrama and Modern Theatre)*. Buenos Aires: La Pleyade.

Fonseca, J. (1980) *Psicodrama da Loucura – Correlações entre Buber e Moreno (The Psychodrama of Madness – Correlations between Buber and Moreno)*. São Paulo: Ágora.

Fonseca, J. (1992) 'Psicodrama ou neopsicodrama?' (Psychodrama or neo-psychodrama?). *Revista Psicodrama* IV, 4, 7–19.

Fonseca, J. (1993) 'As origens do movimento psicodramático Brasileiro' (The beginnings of the Brazilian psychodrama movement). Unpublished interview.

Fonseca, J. (2004) *Contemporary Psychodrama – New Approaches to Theory and Technique*. Hove and New York: Brunner-Routledge.

Freud, S. (1919) 'O "estranho"' (The 'uncanny'). In *The Collected Works of Sigmund Freud*. Rio de Janeiro: Imago, 1969.

Freud, S. (1977) *Dificuldades e Abordagens Iniciais (Initial Difficulties and Approaches)*. Rio de Janeiro: Imago.

GEPSP Bulletin (Bulletins of the São Paulo Psychodrama Study Group). São Paulo, 1968, 1969 and 1970.

Goleman, D. (1996) *La Inteligencia Emocional (Emotional Intelligence)*. Buenos Aires: Javier Vergara.

Gonçalves, C.S. (1988) 'Pequeno comentário sobre a metodologia psicodramática: o lugar da fantasia' (Comments regarding the methodology of psychodrama: a place of fantasy). Paper presented at the sixth Brazilian Psychodrama Conference, Salvador, 1988.

Grimal, P. (1999) *Mitos Gregos e Romanos (Greek and Roman Myths)*. Buenos Aires: Paidós.

Groisman, M., Lobo, M.V. and Cavour, R.M. (1996) *Histórias Dramáticas: Terapia Breve para Famílias e Terapeutas (Dramatic Stories: Brief Therapy for Families and Therapists)*. Rio de Janeiro: Editora Rosa dos Tempos.

Gruspun, H. (1988) *Instituto Sedes Sapientae – 1977-1997 – Histórias e Memórias* (The history and memories of the Sedes Sapientae Institute from 1977 to 1997). Sedes Sapientae Bulletin: São Paulo.

Hammer, E.F. (1978) *Testes Proyectivos Gráficos (Graphic Projective Tests)*. Buenos Aires: Paidós.

Jaspers, K. (1979) *Psicopatologia Geral (General Psychopathology)*. São Paulo: Atheneu.

Kesselman, H. and Pavlovsky, E. (1980) *Clínica Grupal 2. (Clinical Work with Groups)*. Buenos Aires: Busqueda.

Kesselman, H. and Pavlovsky, E. (1989) *A Multiplicação Dramática (The Dramatic Multiplication)*. São Paulo: Hucitec, 1991.

Kesselman, H., Pavlovsky, E. and Frydlewsky L. (1987) 'La obra abierta de Umberto Eco y la multiplicación dramática' (The open composition of Umberto Eco and dramatic multiplication). In E. Pavlovsky *et al. Lo Grupal*. Buenos Aires: Busqueda.

Kesselman, S. and Kesselman, H. (1987) 'Corpodrama' (Corporal-drama). *RAPTG 2*, pp.43–45.

Kroll, J. (1993) *PTSD/Borderlines in Therapy: Finding the Balance*. New York: W.W. Norton and Company Inc.

Laing, R. (1974) *El Yo Dividido (The Divided Ego)*. Buenos Aires: Fondo de Cultura Económica.

Lineham, M.M. (1993) *Cognitive Behavioural Treatment of Borderline Personality Disorder*. New York: Guilford Press.

McGoldrick, M. and Gerson, R. (1985) *Genograms in Family Assessment*. New York: W.W. Norton and Company.

Mahler, M. (1977) *O Nascimento Psicológico Humano (The Psychological Birth of the Human)*. Rio de Janeiro: Zahar.

Marineau, R.F. (1989) *Jacob Levy Moreno, 1889-1974: Father of Psychodrama, Sociometry and Group Psychotherapy*. London and New York: Tavistock/Routledge.

Marques, W.E.U. (2001) *Infâncias (Pre)ocupadas: Trabalho Infantil, Família, Identidade (Worried Childhood: Working with Children, Families and Identity)*. Brasília: Plano.

Martinez Bouquet, C., Moccio, F. and Pavlovsky, E. (1975) *Psicodrama Psicoanalítico en Grupos (Group Psychoanalytic Psychodrama)*. Buenos Aires: Kargieman.

Martins, J.S. (1993) *A Chegada do Estranho (The Arrival of the Stranger)*. São Paulo: Hucitec.

Mascarenhas, P. (1995) 'Multiplicação dramática, uma poética do psicodrama' (Dramatic multiplication, the poetry of psychodrama). Unpublished dissertation, SOPSP/FEBRAP.

Mezher, A. (1980) 'Um questionamento acerca da validade do conceito de papel psicosomático' (An argument around the validity of the concept of psychosomatic roles). *Revista FEBRAP* 3, 1, pp. 221–223.

Miller, A. (1979) *O Drama da Criança bem Dotada (The Drama of the Talented Child)*. São Paulo: Summus.

Millon, T. (1987) 'On the genesis and prevalence of the borderline personality disorder: A social learning thesis'. In M. Lineham (1993) *Cognitive Behavioral Treatment of Borderline Personality Disorder*. New York: Guilford Press.

Montagna, P. (1994) 'Psicanálise e psiquiatria' (Psychoanalysis and psychiatry). In L. Nosek *et al. Album de Família – Imagens, Fontes e Idéias da Psicanálise em São Paulo (Family Album – Images, Sources and Thoughts about Psychoanalysis in São Paulo)*. São Paulo: Casa de Psicólogo.

Moreno, J.L. (1923) *The Theatre of Spontaneity*. New York: Beacon House, 1973.

Moreno, J.L. (1934) *Who Shall Survive? Foundations of Sociometry, Group Psychotherapy and Sociodrama*. New York: Beacon House Inc., 1978.

Moreno, J.L. (1946) *Psychodrama – Volume 1*. New York: Beacon House, 1977.

Moreno, J.L. (1959) *Psychodrama Vol.2. – Foundations of Psychotherapy*. New York: Beacon House, 1975.

Moreno, J.L. (1974) *Psicoterapia de Grupo e Psicodrama (Group Psychotherapy and Psychodrama)*. São Paulo: Mestre Jou.

Moreno, J.L. (1983) *Fundamentos do Psicodrama (Psychodrama, Vol.2. – The Foundations of Psychotherapy)*. São Paulo: Summus.

Munhoz, M. L. (2000) *Casamento: Ruptura ou Continuidade dos Modelos Familiares? (Marriage: Rupture or Continuity of the Family Models?)*. Taubaté: Cabral Editora Universitária.

Nabholtz, A.L.; Capelato, A.; Pierozzi, C.M.; Wolff, M.S.; Montag, N. and Navarro, M.P. (1981) 'A propósito do psicodrama bipessoal' (A proposal for bi-personal psychodrama). *Revista FEBRAP* 4, 1, 35–38.

Naffah Neto, A. (1979) *Psicodrama: Descolonizando o Imaginário (Psychodrama: Decolonizing the Imaginary)*. São Paulo: Brasiliense.

Naffah Neto, A. (1990) *A Paixões e Questões de um Terapeuta (The Passion and Questions of a Therapist)*. São Paulo: Ágora.

Naffah Neto, A. (1995) 'Papel imaginário' (The imaginary role). In C.M. Menegazzo, M.M. Zuretti and M.A. Tomasini *Dicionário de Psicodrama e Sociodrama (The Dictionary of Psychodrama and Sociodrama)*. São Paulo: Ágora, p.151.

Navarro, M.P. *et al.* (1978) 'Mecanismos de ação do psicodrama' (Mechanisms of action in psychodrama). *Revista FEBRAP* 1.

Oliveira, L.L. (1990) *A Socioogia de Guereiro (The Sociology of the Warrior)*. Rio de Janeiro: Editora UFRJ.

Pamplona da Costa, R. (1980) *Videopsicodrama (Video-psychodrama)*. Dissertation presented at the São Paulo Psychodrama Society.

Pamplona da Costa, R. (ed) *(1986) Macho, Masculino, Homem (Macho, Masculinity, Man)*. Porto Alegre: L&PM.

Pavlovsky, E. (1974) *Clinica Grupal (Clinical Work with Groups)*. Buenos Aires: Busqueda.

Pavlovsky, E. (1980) *Espacios y Criatividad (Space and Creativity)*. Buenos Aires: Busqueda.

Pavlovsky, E., Kesselman, H. and Frydlewsky, L. (1978) *La Escenas Temidas del Coordinador de Grupos (Scenes Feared by Group Facilitators)*. Madrid: Fundamentos.

Perazzo, S. (1992) 'Moreno, D. Quixote e a matriz de identidade: uma análise crítica' (Moreno, Don Quixote and the matrix of identity: a critical analysis). In various authors *J.L. Moreno, o Psicodramaturgo (J.L. Moreno, the Psycho-dramaturge)*. São Paulo: Casa do Psicólogo.

Perazzo, S. (1994) *Ainda e Sempre Psicodrama (Psychodrama Still and Forever)*. São Paulo: Ágora.

Perazzo, S. (1995) 'Papel de fantasia' (The fantasy role). In C.M. Menegazzo, M.M. Zuretti and M.A. Tomasini *Dicionário de Psicodrama e Sociodrama (The Dictionary of Psychodrama and Sociodrama)*. São Paulo: Ágora, p.149.

Perazzo, S. (2000) 'Brazil in the psychodrama era.' Leaflet published for the twelfth Brazilian Psychodrama Conference.

Pichon-Riviere, E. (1971) *El Proceso Creador (The Creative Process)*. Buenos Aires: Nueva Vision.

Rocheblave-Spenlé, A.M. (1969) *La Notion de Rôle en Psychologie Sociale (The Notion of Role in Social Psychology)*. Paris: Presses Universitaires de France.

Rodrigues, A. (1977) *Psicologia Social (Social Psychology)*. Rio de Janeiro: Vozes.

Rojas-Bermudez, J.G. (1977) *Introdução ao Psicodrama (Introduction to Psychodrama)*. São Paulo: Editora Mestre Jou.

Rojas-Bermudez, J.G. (1978) *Núcleo do Eu (The Nucleus of the I)*. São Paulo: Natura.

Rojas-Bermudez, J.G. (1984) *Que es el Sicodrama? (What is Psychodrama?)*. Buenos Aires: Celsius.

Rojas-Bermudez, J.R. (1985) *Titeres y Sicodrama (Puppets and Psychodrama)*. Buenos Aires: Celsius.

Rojas-Bermudez, J.R. (1997) *Teoría y Técnica Psicodramáticas (Psychodrama Theory and Technique)*. Barcelona and Buenos Aires: Paidós.

Romaña, M.A. (1989) 'Consideração sobre a esquecida adolescência de J.L. Moreno' (Considerations regarding Moreno's forgotten adolescence). In various authors *J.L. Moreno, o Psicodramaturgo (J.L. Moreno, the Psycho-dramaturge)*. São Paulo: Casa do Psicólogo.

Sampaio, D. and Gameiro, J. (1985) *Terapia Familiar (Family Therapy)*. Porto: Afrontamento.

Santos, A.G. (1989) 'Ação dramática: seu ético e suas roupagens ideológicas (The dramatic action: its ethics and ideological garments). In various authors *J.L. Moreno, o Psicodramaturgo (J.L. Moreno, the Psycho-dramaturge)*. São Paulo: Casa do Psicólogo.

Schutzenberger, A.A. (1997) *Meus Antepassados (My Ancestry)*. São Paulo: Paulus.

Segal, H. (1972) *Introduction to the Work of Melanie Klein*. Buenos Aires: Paidós.

Seixas, M.R. (1992) *Sociodrama Familiar Sistêmico (Systemic Family Sociodrama)*. São Paulo: Aleph.

Smolovich, R. (1985) 'Apuntes sobre multiplicación dramática' (Approaches to dramatic multiplication). In E. Pavlovsky *Lo Grupal*. Buenos Aires: Busqueda.

Souza Leite, M.P. (1977) 'Enfoque psicodramático das psicoses, núcleo do eu' (Psychodramatic focus in psychosis, the nucleus of the I). *Temas* VII, 13, 125–137.

Velho, G. (1986) *Subjetividade e Sociedade, uma Experiência de Geração (Subjectivity and Society: A Generational Experience)*. Rio de Janeiro: Zahar.

Ventura, Z. (1998) *O Mal Secreto (The Secret Evil)*. Buenos Aires: Objective Ltda.

Vitale, M.A.F. (1994) 'Vergonha: um estudo em três gerações (Shame: a study in three generations). PhD dissertation, PUC-SP.

Vitale, M.A.F. (1999) 'Separação e ciclo vital familiar: um enfoque sociodramático' (Separation and the family life cycle: a sociodramatic focus) In W.C. Almeida *Grupos: a Proposta do Psicodrama (Groups: A Psychodramatic Proposal)*. São Paulo, Ágora.

Vitale, M.A.F. (2003) 'Avós novas e velhas figuras da família contemporânea' (Young and old grandparents within the contemporary family). In R.A. Acosta and M.A.F. *Vitale Família: Redes, Laços e Políticas Públicas (The family: Networks, Relationships and Public Politics)*. São Paulo: IEE PUC-SP.

Volpe, A.J. (1990) *Édipo: Psicodrama do Destino (Oedipus: The Psychodrama of Destiny)*. São Paulo: Ágora.

Watzlawick, P., Beavin, J.H. and Jackson, D.D. (1981) *Pragmática da Comunicação Humana (The Pragmatism of Human Communication)*. São Paulo: Cultrix.

Weil, P. (1967) *Psicodrama (Psychodrama)*. Rio de Janeiro: Cepa.

Willi, J. (1978) *La Pareja Humana: Relación y Conflicto (The Human Couple: Relationship and Conflict)*. Madrid: Morate.

Williams, A. (1989) *The Passionate Technique: Strategic Psychodrama with Individuals, Families and Groups*. London and New York: Routledge.

Wolff, J.R.A.S. (1981) 'Onirodrama – contribuição ao estudo dos sonhos em psicoterapia psicodramática' (Onirodrama – The study of dreams and psychodrama psychotherapy). Dissertation presented at the São Paulo Medical School.

Wolff, J.R. (1985) *Sonho e Loucura (Dream and Madness)*. São Paulo: Ática.

Zimmermann, D. (1971) 'Estudos sobre psicoterapia analítica de grupo' (Study about group analytical psychotherapy). In *Esboço Histórico da Psicoterapia Analítica de Grupo no Brasil (A Historical Sketch of the Brazilian Group Analytical Psychotherapy)*. São Paulo: Mestre Jou.

Contributors

Moysés Aguiar is a psychologist, psycho- and sociotherapist, spontaneity theatre director; psychodrama trainer and supervisor with the Brazilian Psychodrama Federation (FEBRAP); coordinator of the 'Companhia do Teatro Espontâneo' (Spontaneous Theatre Ensemble), a project for experimental spontaneous theatre ensemble and training.

Luis Altenfelder is a psychiatrist and psychodramatist; psychodrama trainer, supervisor and didactic therapist at the Brazilian Psychodrama Federation (FEBRAP); director of the Psycho-social Rehabilitation Centre of the Clinicas Hospital.

Dalmiro M. Bustos is a psychiatrist and psychodramatist; director of the J.L. Moreno Psychodrama Institutes in Buenos Aires and São Paulo; supervisor and trainer at the São Paulo Psychodrama Society.

Rosa Cukier is a psychologist; psychoanalyst; psychodramatist; trainer-supervisor at the São Paulo Psychodrama Society (SOPSP) and the São Paulo Moreno Institute; psychotherapist.

Luís Falivene R. Alves is a physician and psychiatrist, psychodramatist at the São Paulo Psychodrama Society (SOPSP) and the J.L. Moreno Institute (São Paulo); therapist and supervisor at the Brazilian Psychodrama Federation (FEBRAP); trainer and supervisor at the Campinas Psychodrama and Group Psychotherapy Institute (IPPGC).

Antonio Ferrara is a psychodramatist; director of the São Paulo Playback Theatre Company.

Zoltán Figusch is a clinical and educational psychologist; psychodrama psychotherapist registered with the British Psychodrama Association (BPA) and the United Kingdom Council of Psychotherapists (UKCP); associate member of the São Paulo Psychodrama Society (SOPSP). After living in Brazil for two years, he has recently returned to the UK and works as a psychodrama psychotherapist in Manchester. He can be contacted through e-mail: figusch@hotmail.com

José Fonseca, PhD, is a psychiatrist and psychotherapist; psychodrama trainer and supervisor at the São Paulo Psychodrama Society (SOPSP); coordinator of the DAIMON Centre for Relationship Studies in São Paulo; former editor of the International FORUM of Group Psychotherapy.

Sonia Marmelsztejn is a psychologist; psychodramatist; psychotherapist.

Pedro Mascarenhas is a psychiatrist, psychoanalyst and psychodramatist; trainer and supervisor at the São Paulo Psychodrama Association (SOPSP) and the Brazilian Psychodrama Federation (FEBRAP).

Geraldo Massaro is a psychiatrist and psychodramatist; psychodrama trainer and supervisor at the Sedes Sapientae Institute, the Paulista Psychodrama Society (SOVAP) and the Psychiatry Institute of the São Paulo Medical School (IPqHCFMUSP).

Ronaldo Pamplona da Costa is a psychiatrist; therapist; psychodrama trainer and supervisor at the São Paulo Psychodrama Society (SOPSP); sexology trainer and therapist; researcher in video-psychodrama and tele-psychodrama.

Sergio Perazzo is a psychiatrist, psychodramatist; trainer-supervisor at the São Paulo Psychodrama Society (SOPSP) and the São Paulo Catholic University (PUC).

Maria Amalia Faller Vitale, PhD, is a psychodramatist and family therapist; psychodrama trainer and teacher at the Post-Graduate Social Services Programme of the São Paulo Catholic University; coordinator of the Family Therapy Course at the Psychiatric Unit of the Paulista Medical School.

Subject index

Page entries marked with an 'n' refer to the notes at the end of chapters.

abandonment 97–8, 102, 107, 110, 205
abuse 112, 207, 212, 214, 224
　emotional 207
　physical 207
　sexual 112, 207
'act hunger' 97
acting out, irrational 174
action 152, 172
　dramatic 152–3, 172
actor 125, 127, 152
　therapeutic 252
adequacy (as ego function) 93, 106
'admiration' 102
adolescence/adolescents 44
affirmation in therapy 214
aggression 106–7, 112–13, 119
alarm state/alertness 75, 83, 86
　acute 83
　chronic 83
anger 100, 203, 205, 214, 218
　concretization of 223–4
anti-psychiatry model 200
　see also psychiatry movement in São Paulo
anxiety 99–100, 106
area(s) 77–8
　body 77–8, 81–2
　confusion 80–2
　environment 77–8, 81–2
　integration, the theory of 37, 73
　mind 77–8, 81–2
Argentinean Psychodrama Association 28, 30, 32
art 154–6
　analytical art therapy 171
'as if' 139, 148
asymmetric roles 50, 109–10, 120
atogram/action diagram 180
audience 152, 200, 255–6, 266
　second 252, 254, 260, 262
　television 265–8
　test 251
authority 111, 225
autonomy 96, 109, 112

auxiliary ego 255–8

Barbara case (Moreno) 178, 188n
basic ontological insecurity 97
beliefs 186
Bermudian psychodrama 17, 24–32, 37–40, 57, 71–89, 173
body 72, 97
　area 77–8, 81–2
borderline personality disorder 203–26
boundaries 204, 214, 215, 216
　of the self 74–5, 83, 86, 173
　see also 'nucleus of the I' theory
Brazilian Association of Analytical Group Psychotherapy 24
Brazilian Journal of Psychodrama 39
Brazilian Psychoanalytic Society 19, 27
　see also psychoanalytic movement in São Paulo 18–22
Brazilian psychodrama conferences 39
Brazilian Psychodrama Federation (FEBRAP) 32, 39, 64
Brazilian psychodrama movement 36–9, 64–7
　identity 48, 55–60, 63–7
　pioneers 22–5, 33, 46
　training 27–32, 57
　see also São Paulo Psychodrama Study Group
Brazilian Psychodrama and Sociodrama Association (ABPS) 32, 38
breast feeding 95

Cain and Abel 101, 115
cannibalism 53
　cultural 54
carnival 123
catechesis 52
catharsis of integration 148, 174, 199
causal chain 148

choice(s), sociometric 179, 230–3, 234–5
　incongruence 232
　mutuality 232
　negative 230–3, 234–5
　neutral/indifferent (or neutrality) 230–1, 234–5
　positive 230–3, 234–5
　see also sociometry
Christ archetype 117
cinema 250, 267
cluster(s) 90–121
　effect 91, 93
　fraternal (or cluster three) 114–18
　maternal (or cluster one) 95–108
　paternal (or cluster two) 108–14
　theory (or role theory) 90–121
co-being, matrix of identity 91
co-conscious states 139, 179
co-experience, matrix of identity 91
colonization 51–8, 60–3
　primary 55–9
　role of the colonized 48, 51–5, 60–3
　role of the colonizer 48, 51–5, 60–3
　secondary 55–9
comments and analysis, the phase of 116, 146
communication 174, 228–9
　theory 191, 227–8
competition 116–17
complementary roles 50, 52, 74–5, 92, 123–4
compulsive actions 82, 206
concretization
　of anger 223–4
　technique of 161–5, 174
conferences
　Brazilian psychodrama 39
　group psychotherapy, international 58
　group psychotherapy, Latin-American 21, 23, 24, 26
　psychodrama conference in São Paulo, international 30–1, 38
　psychodrama and sociodrama, international 25, 28, 29

280

SUBJECT INDEX

confidentiality 252, 258
control 112
convulsive therapy 19
cooling down the protagonist 220
co-responsibility 50, 56
corporal drama 195
corporal memory 94, 97
corporal zones in interaction 41, 129n
co-unconscious 139, 179
counter-culture 63
couple therapy 175–89, 259
creation 150–6
  co-creation 153
  collective/group 134, 150–1, 193–4, 202
creative matrix 194
criterion/criteria, sociometric 109, 141, 230
  see also sociometry
cultural atom 180
cultural conserve 57, 250
cultural norms and values 49, 52, 124
cultural product 61–3
cycloid personality 225

defecator
  model 79
  role 49, 77–83, 92
  see also psychosomatic roles and models
defence mechanisms 75, 83, 98–9
delirium 83–4, 126, 174
denial 101
dependence/dependency 55, 95–6, 99, 209
depression 82, 107
development 48–51, 72–3, 155
  see also emotional development; psychological development
development theory 37, 41
developmental phases 91–121
diagnosis 143–5, 171
diagnostic psychodrama 143–5
diathesis 80–1
director 139, 143, 255
  role 150
  video- 254–9
dissociation 99, 207
double technique 160, 220
drama 42

dramatic
  action 152–3, 172
  context 130–40, 147–50, 255
multiplication
  concept 190–2
  technique 190–200
project 141–2
roles 124–8
dramatization 154, 159–61, 172, 174
drawings 159–74
dream technique (onirodrama) 44, 161

ego 92–3, 98
electroshock therapy 198
elements of psychodrama, the 255
emission index 227, 236–48
emitter 228
  faulty 229, 236–39
  see also perceptive test
empathy 214, 217
emotion(s) 94, 208–9
  primary/basic 96, 100–2
emotional development 207, 210
emotional intelligence 94
emotional skin 208
emotional survival 97
environment 76
  area 77–8, 81–2
envy 100–2
  healthy/creative 102
ethics 258
existentialism 144
existential emptiness 206
existential phenomenology 42

family 175–89, 207–9
  history 177, 187
  life cycle 175–6, 186
  primary 176, 188n, 198
  sociometric network 175–6
  therapy 175–89, 259
fantastic roles 126–7
fantasy
  and reality, breach between 49, 72, 109, 126
  roles 49, 129n
father 93, 108–14
  father–child relationship 93, 109, 113

see also paternal cluster; paternal function
first universe 126
focus 141–4
fraternal cluster (or cluster three) 114–20

genetic structures (*see also* the 'nucleus of the I' theory)
  externally programmed 76, 80
  internally programmed 76, 80
genodrama 175–89
  technique of 182–8
genogram 175–89
Gestalt 145–7
  psychodrama 145–7
  theory 145
  therapy 145–7
god(s) 115
  Greek 101
gratitude 102
Greek
  chorus 136, 138, 140
  gods 102
  tragedy 136, 138, 140, 151
grounding 109, 112
group
  context 130–40, 255
  representative 138–9
Group of Eleven, the 31
guilt 102–5
guilt–punishment equation 103

hallucination 174
holding 108
horizontal approach in psychodrama 147
hysteria, phobic 81–2
hysteric conversion 81–2
hysteric syndromes 172

idealization 204, 209
identity 205–8
  of Brazilian psychodrama 48, 55–60, 63–7
  double 54
  matrix of all 43, 48–50, 71–2, 91–3, 95, 100
  see also matrix of identity
imaginary roles 40, 49, 126–9
  non-transferential 129n
  transferential 129n
imagination 153–4
improvisation 152, 193

impulsivity 206
incorporation 54
incorporative mechanisms 83
incorporative–eliminatory phase of development 50–3
index of group tele 227, 236–49
    see also perceptive test
individualism 62, 117, 208
individualization 181
individual psychodrama 38, 40, 259
indoctrination 52
ingestor model 79
    see also psychosomatic roles and models
ingestor role 49, 77–83, 124
insight, psychodramatic 168, 174
instincts 105
instruments of psychodrama 130
interaction 49, 93, 124–5
internalization 92
International Association of Group Psychotherapy (IAGP) 24
International Psychoanalytic Association (IPA) 19
intermediary object 76, 85–9, 89n, 173
intermediary situation 89n
interpersonal intelligence 94
interpolation of metaphors, technique 223–4
interview of a character, technique 144–5, 161
    initial 177
intrusive–receptive phase of development 50–3

jealousy 111–2
joint creation 134, 150–1, 193–4, 202
Judas 101
Juqueri Hospice 18, 27

Karl, the case of (or the psychodrama of Adolf Hitler) 196–202

language 201–2, 265
latent roles 49
leader role 111
links/linking 74–5, 86, 174
    see also 'nucleus of the I' theory

Macunaima 54, 59n
machine 191–2
malpractice 217
mania 83
marital/conjugal relationship 175–89
mass therapy 252
maternal cluster (or cluster one) 95–108
maternal function 92, 95–105
matrix of identity 43, 48–50, 71–2, 91–5, 100, 126
    theory 41
melancholy 83
memory trace 76, 80
mental illness 80
military dictatorship/regime 28, 30, 253
mind area 77–8, 81–2
mirror, technique 160–2, 221–2
modes and modalities of roles 50–3
molar view 153
molecular view 153, 198
monocular perspective 194, 198
mother 91, 95–105, 124
    internal 106
    mother–child relationship 92, 109, 113
    see also maternal cluster; maternal function
mutism 83
myths 92, 98

needs 76, 80, 92–3, 99
    biological 92
    physiological 80
negativism 83
negotiation 118–19
neo-psychodrama 44
neurosis 82, 204
neutrality 230–1, 234–5
    see also sociometric choices
'nucleus of the I' 76–80
    theory 37, 71–89

objective test, sociometry 231, 234, 244
obsessive ideas and thoughts 82
occupied/occupant 60–3
oppression/oppressor 37
organizational psychodrama 251
Othello and Iago 101, 112
overprotection 98, 105

parental relationship 114
partial self 72, 88n
paternal cluster (or cluster two) 108–14
paternal function 93, 108–14
pathetic, concept 194, 200, 202
perception 145–7, 227
perceptive structures 146
perceptive test 227–49
    emission index 227, 236–48
    graphic representation of the perceptive test 233–40
    index of group tele 227, 236–49
    perception index 227, 236–48
    tabular representation of the perceptive test 240–49
    tele index 227, 236–49
permission, concept 216
personal role 125–8
personality 73
    traces 144
phenomenology 42
phobic symptoms 81–2, 161
physiological mechanisms/functions 76
physiological self 72, 77–8
physio-psychopathology 80–5
pioneers of Brazilian psychodrama 22–5, 33, 46
play/playful 193–4, 200
playback theatre 152
pleasure 96
plot 131, 150
porosity 80–1
    see also psychosomatic roles
power 52, 62–3, 103
pragmatic psychodrama 149–50
processing, the phase of 257–8
projection 101, 171
    projective test 171
protagonist 42, 130–40 255
    cooling down 220
    pre-/intermediary 139
protagonic theme 130–9
protoroles 92
psychiatric/medical model 144
    see also psychiatry movement in São Paulo
psychiatry movement in São Paulo 18–22
psychoanalytic courses in São Paulo 19
psychoanalytic movement in São Paulo 18–22
psycho-cameraman 255

SUBJECT INDEX

psychodrama of Adolf Hitler (or
  The case of Karl) 196–202
Psychodrama Remembrance
  Project 17, 33
psychodrama, street 65, 254
psychodrama training in São
  Paulo 27–32, 57
psychodramatic insight 168, 174
psychodramatic roles 40, 49, 72,
  126–8
psycho-dramaturge 45
psychogram, the technique of
  159–74
psychological development 49,
  71
psychopathic personality 82,
  107, 147
psychopathology
  psychodramatic 41, 143–5
  theory 37
  see also
    physio-psychopathology
psychosis 82–4, 180, 197–8,
  204, 206
  spatial 84, 89n
  temporal 84, 89n
psychosomatic models 79
psychosomatic roles 37, 41, 49,
  72–3, 76–81, 92, 124,
  142
  defecator 49, 77–83, 92
  ingestor 49, 77–83, 123
  urinator 49, 77–83, 92
  see also 'nucleus of the I'
    theory
psychotic behaviour 82
psychotic clients 76, 85, 174
Ptono (Greek god of envy) 101
public psychodrama 24–7, 57,
  261
puppets and marionettes 76, 85

reality, protagonist 154–5
receiver 228
  faulty 229, 236–9
  see also perceptive test
recognition of the I 41, 50, 160
recognition of the other 41, 50
regressive psychodrama 148
relationship 48–55, 96, 204,
  227
  asymmetric 50, 109–10, 120
  interpersonal, theory 91
  psychotherapeutic 183–4

symmetric 50, 114–20
  therapeutic 210–12, 218
religion
  fundamentalism 115
  rituals 136
  values 52
reparatory mechanisms 81–2
reparatory psychodrama 147–9
repression 99
resistance 106
resonance 193, 201
  transpersonal 193
responsibility 103–4, 119, 153
rivalry 115–18
roles
  apparent 49
  asymmetric 50, 109–10, 120
  atom 180
  clusters 90–121
    see also cluster(s)
  colonized 48, 51–5, 60–3
  colonizer 48, 51–5, 60–3
  complementarity 50, 52,
    74–5, 92, 123
  creating 57
  development 75
  reversal, technique 160, 224
  structure 49, 73–6, 80, 173
  taking 57
  taking the role of the other,
    the technique of 160,
    164
  theory 40–1, 48–51, 71–3,
    122–29
  of clusters, the 90–121
role-play/role-playing 49, 57,
  149, 251

São Paulo
  Psychoanalytical Group 20
  Psychoanalytical Society 20–2
  Psychodrama Society (SOSPS)
    32, 38
  Psychodrama Study Group
    (GEPSP) 27–32
  Society of Psychology and
    Group Psychotherapy 26
scene 128–9, 191
  nodal 148
schizo-analysis 191, 201, 202,
  202n
script 131, 152
second universe 126
Sedes Sapientae Institute 17,
  20–3, 27

self 72–3, 204
  partial 72, 88n
self-confidence 111
self-destructive/self-harming
  behaviour 206–7, 225
self-esteem 97, 101, 205
semiotics 201–2, 265
shame 104–6
sharing
  as a dynamic of cluster three
    115–17
  as a phase of psychodrama 38,
    116, 146, 193
  through action 193–8
siblings 93, 114–18
  fraternal cluster (or cluster
    three) 114–18
social atom 73, 83, 174, 180,
  189n
social context 58, 71, 131, 137,
  148–50, 255
social placenta 72
social psychoanalysis 192
social roles 49, 72–4, 123–8
sociatry 267
society 72, 93
sociodrama 131, 152, 196–8
  family 187
sociogram 179–80
  geno-sociogram 180
sociometric character types 229
sociometric choice 179, 230–1,
  234–5
sociometric criteria 109, 141,
  230
sociometric test 141, 179, 227,
  230–3
sociometry 109, 227–49
socionomic project 40
soliloquy, technique 160
spectator 262
spontaneism 93
spontaneity 57, 93, 99, 105, 150
  and creativity theory 40
  training 149
spontaneous/creative state
  193–5, 201
spontaneous theatre 141–56
stage 152, 255
submission 52, 112
subordination 55
suicide 203, 206
  para-suicidal behaviour 206,
    225n
supervision 258

surplus reality, technique 222
symbolization, technique 161
symmetric roles 50, 114–20
systemic approach 177–8
systems theory 178

tele 42, 189n, 227, 239
　index 227, 236–49
　index of group 227, 236–49
tele-psychodrama 250–69
　pedagogical 263
tele-relationship 229, 239
television 250, 252, 267
　closed circuit 260–2
　open 262–7
tenderness 96–7, 108
theatre 126, 142, 150–2
　Greek 136, 138, 140, 151
　of spontaneity 141–56
　therapeutic 42, 130
théatre reciproque 178
therapeutic context 132
therapeutic films 250–2, 267
therapist role 108, 112, 120
third parent 114
trans-individuality 193
transitional zone 194
trauma 147–8
triadic psychodrama 25
truth, Morenian 198

uncanny 194, 200, 202
unconscious 105, 171–3, 191
　collective 98, 105
　see also co-unconscious
under-developed roles 74–5, 86
undifferentiated world 77
urinator
　model 79
　role 49, 77–83, 92
　see also psychosomatic roles
　　and models

validation 214, 216, 225
vertical approach in psychodrama
　147
video-director 254–9
video-psychodrama 250–67
　on CCTV 260–2
　context 255
　Group of Experimental
　　Video-Psychodrama, the
　　253
　on open television 262–7
　pedagogical 263
　in therapy 254–60
violence 52, 112
voracity 100
vulnerability of the therapist 216

warm-up 75, 85, 174, 260, 262
　audience 266
well developed roles 74
World Centre of Psychodrama,
　Sociometry and Group
　Psychotherapy 28–9, 32

Author index

Aeschylus 136
Aguiar, M. 42–5, 141–57
Almeida, W.C. 42, 190, 201
Altenfelder, L. 89n, 159–76
Andrade, M. 55, 59n
Anzieu, D. 192
Azevedo, I. S. 22–7, 31

Bicudo, V. 19–20
Bion, W. 192
Blatner, H. 172
Blay Neto, B. 23
Borba, C. 17, 33, 254, 263–5
Bour, P. 89n
Bowen, M. 177
Brecht, B. 151
Bustos, D.M. 38, 57, 90–121, 172, 228–40

Campedelli, A.M. 40
Castro, F. 117
Cesarino, A.C. 24, 26–7, 31–2
Churchill, W. 197
Cukier, R. 46n, 58, 203–26

D'Alessandro, J.M. 23, 25, 27, 29, 31
D'Andrea, F.F. 22–4
Deleuze, G. 191, 195, 202n
Dias, F. 19
Dias Reis, M. 46n
Di Loreto, O. 25–6
Dolto, F. 187

Echanis, J. 28
Eco, U. 190–1, 201
Euripides 136
Eva, A.C. 26

Falivene Alves, L. 42, 130–40, 225
Fanchette, J. 147
Fenichel, O. 19
Ferrara, A. 227–49
Figusch, Z. 71–89

Fonseca, J. 26, 32, 40–1, 44, 46n, 48–59, 127–8, 183–4, 253
Foulkes, S.H. 192–5
Franco da Rocha, F. 18–19
Freud, A. 98
Freud, S. 172, 192, 194
Frydlewsky, L. 190–2

Gaiarsa, J.A. 253
Garcia, C. 18, 22–4
Goebbels, J. 196
Goering 196–9
Goleman, D. 192
Gonçalves, C. S. 44
Greeb, M. 32
Gruspun, H. 23
Guattari, F. 191, 195, 202n
Guevara, C. 55

Jaspers, K. 160, 172
Jatoba, N. 23
Jones, E. 19

Kaufman, A. 46n
Kesselman, H. 190–5
Kesselman, S. 192, 195
Klein, M. 98, 100, 102
Kleinberg, O. 22, 33n
Knobel, A. M. 46n, 58
Koch, A. 19–20
Kroll, J. 212, 217

Lacan, J. 201
Laing, R.D. 97
Lebovici, S. 192
Lineham, M.M. 203, 212, 218
Lopes, L. 32

Macondes, D. 18–9, 21
Marineau, R. 178
Marmelsztejn, S. 203–26
Martins, C. 25
Martins, J. S. 53–5
Mascarenhas, P. 45, 190–200
Massaro, G. 46n, 60–7
Mazieres, G. 29
Merengue, D. 46n
Mezher, A. 26, 41, 123–5
Miller, A. 226

Millon, T. 225
Monteiro, R. 253–6
Moreira, U. 31–2
Moreno, J.L. 28–9, 31–2, 250
Moreno, Z. 27, 41, 147
Mother Christina (Sister Celia Sodre Doria) 17, 20, 23
Munhoz, M.L. 175, 188n
Mussolini 197

Naffah Neto, A. 40–3, 49, 122–8, 200
Navarro, M. P. 26, 46n, 160

Pacheco e Silva, A.C. 18–9, 21, 25
Pamplona da Costa, R. 17–34, 250–67
Pavlovsky, E. 179, 190–5
Perazzo, S. 35–47, 49, 122–9
Perls, F. 146
Piaget, J. 155
Pichon-Riviere, E. 37, 40, 73, 192, 194
Pines, M. 192
Porto, L. 24

Ramos, G. 22
Renones, A.V. 46n
Rocheblave-Spenle, A.M. 41, 122–9
Rojas-Bermudez, J. 17, 24–32, 37–40, 57, 71–89, 173
Romana, M. A. 29, 32, 44, 46n
Roosevelt, F. 197

Salvador, V. 53
Santos, A.G. 36, 122
Schutzenberger, A.A. 25, 180
Seixas, M. 58, 178
Slavson, R.S. 192
Smolovich, R. 195
Socrates 101
Soeiro, A. 23, 25, 27, 31, 46n
Sonenreich, C. 26
Souza Leite, M.P. 39
Stalin 197
Stern, A. 203
Swartzchild, M. 26–7

Thespis 136
Tiba, I. 32

Uchoa, D.M. 25

Vampre, E. 19
Vitale, M.A.F. 175–89
Volpe, J.A. 42

Watzlawick, P. 228
Wechsler, M.P.F. 46n
Weil, P. 17, 21–5, 32, 57
Williams, A. 147
Winnicott, D. 193–4
Wolff, J.R. 44